TEXTBOOK OF
METALLIC STENTS

TEXTBOOK OF METALLIC STENTS

Edited by

Andreas Adam MB BSc(Hons) MRCP FRCP FRCR
Professor, Division of Radiological Sciences, Guy's and St Thomas' Medical and
Dental School, St Thomas' Street, London, England

Robert F. Dondelinger MD
Professor of Radiology at the University of Liège, Head of the Department of
Medical Imaging, University Hospital Sart Tilman, Liège, Belgium

Peter R. Mueller MD
Associate Professor of Radiology, Division Head, Abdominal Imaging and
Interventional Radiology, Massachusetts General Hospital and Harvard Medical
School, Boston, USA

I S I S
MEDICAL
MEDIA
—
Oxford

British Library Cataloguing in Publication Data
A catalogue record for this title is available from the British Library

ISBN   1 899066 32 2

Adam, A (Andreas)
Textbook of Metallic Stents/
Andreas Adam, Robert F. Dondelinger, Peter R. Mueller (eds)

Always refer to the manufacturer's Prescribing Information
before prescribing drugs cited in this book

Typeset by
Creative Associates Ltd, Oxford, UK

Printed by
Dah Hua Printing Press Co. Ltd., Hong Kong

Distributed by
Times Mirror International Publishers
Customer Service Centre, Unit 1, 3 Sheldon Way
Larkfield, Aylesford, Kent ME20 6SF, UK

Contents

List of Contributors

Andreas Adam MB BSc(Hons) FRCP FRCR
Professor, Division of Radiological Sciences, Guy's and St Thomas' Medical and Dental School, St Thomas' Street, London SE1 9RT, England

Karl Barange MD
Service de Gastroenterologie, CHU Purpan, 31054 Toulouse, France

Heinrich D. Becker MD OA
Thorax Klinik der LVA-Baden, Amalienstrasse 5, 69126 Heidelberg-Rohrbach, Germany

Giles W. Boland MD
Department of Radiology, Massachusetts General Hospital and Harvard Medical School, Fruit Street, Boston, MA 02114, USA

Irene Boos MD
Department of Radiodiagnosis and Nuclear Medicine, EV. Diakonissenkrankenhaus, Karlsruhe-Ruppurr, 76199, Karlsruhe, Germany

Patrizio Capasso MD
Staff Radiologist, Co-Director, Section of Interventional Radiology, Department of Radiology, University Hospital Lausanne, Switzerland

Robert F. Dondelinger MD
Professor of Radiology at the University of Liège, Head of Department of Medical Imaging, University Hospital Sart Tilman B35, Liège, Belgium

Joe El-Khoury MD
Service de Radiologie, CHU Rangueil, 1, avenue Jean Poulhes, 31054 Toulouse, France

Rolf W. Guenther MD
Professor, Department of Diagnostic Radiology, Technical University of Aachen, Pauwelsstrasse 30, 52057 Aachen, Germany

Francis Joffre
Professor, Service de Radiologie, CHU Rangueil, 1, avenue Jean Poulhes, 31054 Toulouse, Cedex, France

Barry T. Katzen MD FACR FACC
Medical Director, Miami Vascular Institute at Baptist Hospital; Professor of Clinical Radiology, Department of Radiology, University of Miami School of Medicine, 8900 N. Kendall Drive, Miami, FL 33176, USA

Dieter Liermann
Consultant Radiologist, Zentrum der Radiologie, Klinikum J.W. Goethe Universität, Theodor Stern Kai 7, 60590 Frankfurt am Main, Germany

Pierre Maquin MD
Service de Radiologie, CHU Rangueil, 1, avenue Jean Poulhes, 31054 Toulouse, France

Robert C. Mason
Senior Lecturer in Surgery, Department of Surgery, UMDS, Guy's Hospital, London SE1 9RT, England

Klaus D. Mathias
Professor of Diagnostic Radiology and Neuroradiology, Head of Department, Instituts fü-r Strahlendiagnostik, Stadische Kliniken Dortmund, Beurhausstrasse 40, 44137 Dortmund, Germany

Euan J. G. Milroy FRCS
Consultant Urologist, 77 Harley Street, London NW1, England

Peter R. Mueller MD
Associate Professor of Radiology, Division Head, Abdominal Imaging and Interventional Radiology, Massachusetts General Hospital and Harvard Medical School, Fruit Street, Boston, MA 02144, USA

Brian L. Murphy MD
Department of Radiology, Massachusetts General Hospital and Harvard Medical School, Fruit Street, Boston, MA 02144, USA

Philippe Otal MD
Service de Radiologie, CHU Rangueil, 1, avenue Jean Poulhes, 31054 Toulouse, France

David Rickards MRCS FFRDSA FRCR
Consultant Uroradiologist, Department of Radiology, The Middlesex Hospital, Mortimer Street, London W1N 8AA, England

Hervé Rousseau
Professor, Service de Radiologie, CHU Rangueil, 1, avenue Jean Poulhes, 31054 Toulouse, France

Michael Rust MD OA
Department of Pneumology and Gastroenterology, Klinikum J. W. Goethe Universität, Theodor Stern Kai, 60590 Frankfurt am Main, Germany

Hans H. Schild MD PhD
Professor of Radiology, Director and Chairman, Radiologische Universitätsklinik, Sigmund-Freud Strasse 25, 53105 Bonn, Germany

Ernst-Peter Strecker
Professor of Radiology, Department of Radiodiagnosis and Nuclear Medicine, Ev. Diakonissenkrankenhaus, Karlsruhe-Ruppurr, 76199 Karlsruhe, Germany

Holger Strunk MD PhD
Oberarzt, Radiologische Universitätsklinik, Sigmund-Freud Strasse 25, 53105 Bonn, Germany

Tino Tancredi MD
Specialist Resident, Section of Abdominal Imaging, Department of Medical Imaging University Hospital Sart Tilman, B35, Liège, Belgium

Geneviève Trotteur MD
Chief, Section of Vascular and Interventional Imaging, Department of Medical Imaging, University Hospital Sart Tilman, B35, Liège, Belgium

Jean-Pierre Vinel
Professor, Service d'Hépato-Gastroenterologie du CHU de Toulouse, 31054 Toulouse, France

Dierk Vorwerk MD
Professor of Radiology, Department of Diagnostic Radiology, Technical University of Aachen, Pauwelsstrasse 30, 52057 Aachen, Germany

Anthony Watkinson BSc MSc(Oxon) MBBS FRCS FRCR
Consultant and Honarary Senior Lecturer in Radiology, X-Ray Department, Royal Free Hospital, Pond Street, London NW3, England

Preface

When metallic stents were first introduced many interventional radiologists, and even more medical practitioners in other specialties, thought that they represented a passing fashion. During the last decade developments in this field have been both rapid and substantial. These devices now have an established role in the treatment of many conditions, and the indications for their use are constantly increasing. The first widespread application of metallic stents was in the management of patients with malignant obstructive jaundice, who have a relatively short life expectancy and in whom occlusion of the stent does not have catastrophic consequences. However, stents are now being used in conditions such as aortic aneurysms and carotid stenosis — an illustration of increasing confidence accompanied by technical advance.

The development of metallic stents is still at a very early stage. The devices produced by various manufacturers tend to be based on a single basic design which is then applied to endoprostheses of various sizes for a variety of applications. This situation is likely to change: in future designs will emerge which are more precisely adapted to the anatomy and physiology of the condition being treated. Coatings of various types, variations in calibre at different points within the same stent, a wider choice in the radial force being exerted by the device, and other advances, are likely to ensure that metallic endoprostheses make an increasing contribution in modern medicine.

This textbook, written by contributors at the forefront of this field, describes the major current applications of metallic endoprostheses. Such is the pace of change that the book is likely to become outdated very rapidly. However, we hope that it will provide essential information for clinical work and research, and provide a stimulus for new developments.

A. Adam
R.F. Dondelinger
P.R. Mueller

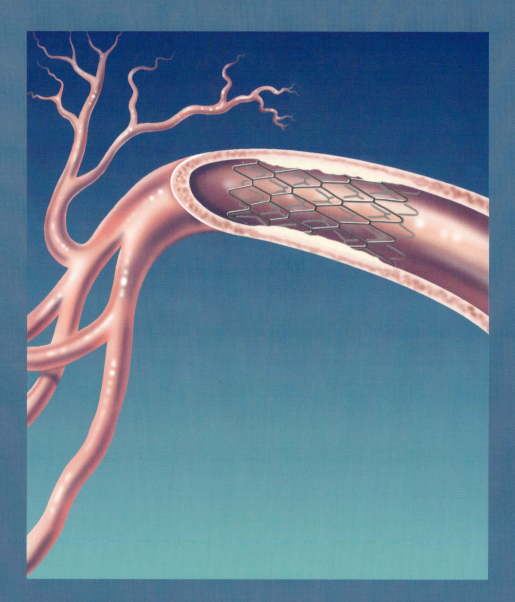

Chapter 1
Arterial stent placement

D. Vorwerk and R.W. Guenther

Introduction

Vascular endoluminal endoprostheses were introduced in the late 1980s and became a valuable new technique for interventional radiologists and cardiologists. While there has been an increase in the number of indications for the insertion of vascular endoprostheses, the most important uses are in stenotic vessels and the management of complications of balloon angioplasty.

Early enthusiasm was enormous but has decreased recently since follow-up results revealed that, although a number of problems can be solved by this new technique, an even larger number of problems remain that cannot be overcome by arterial stents. The main problem is extensive neointimal growth within the stents leading to restenosis or rethrombosis.

A number of different stents have been used in peripheral arterial vessels. The Wallstent™ (Schneider, AG, Bulach, Switzerland), Palmaz™ (Johnson & Johnson, Warren, NJ, USA) and Strecker® (Boston Scientific Inc., Watertown, MA, USA) stents are the most common, and have been described in reports with long-term follow-up (Fig. 1.1). Newer stent devices, the Nitinol Memotherm™ (Angiomed–Bard, Karlsruhe, Germany) stent (Fig. 1.1(b)) and the Cragg stent (MinTec, Freeport, Grand Bahama), have not yet been studied over long periods of time.

Figure 1.1
(a) Wallstent, Strecker stent and Palmaz stent (from above). (b) Nitinol Memotherm stent.

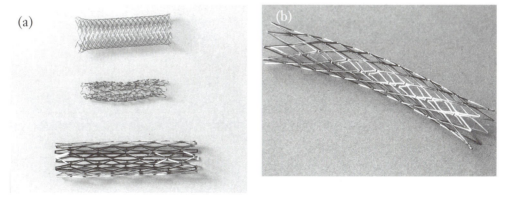

Indications for arterial stenting

General remarks

There are only a few primary indications for stenting. The type and morphology of the lesion, the outcome of balloon angioplasty and the presence or absence of complications, are important criteria in deciding on the placement of a stent. This is particularly true for treatment for restenosis. For example, there is as yet no proof that stent placement is more effective than successful balloon angioplasty in prevention of restenosis. Similarly, there is no proof that in a restenosed vessel use of a stent would be successful in preventing recurrent stenosis.

Aorta and iliac arteries

Becker and co-workers compiled percutaneous transluminal angioplasty (PTA) data for aortoiliac balloon angioplasty from a number of reports describing 2679 procedures;[1] these indicated an average technical success of 92%, a 2-year patency of 81% (range 65–93%) and a 5-year patency of 72% (range 50–87%). Recent advances in catheter and wire technology have contributed to improved results with this technique. Gardiner and co-workers described a total complication rate of 4.5% and a major complication rate requiring surgery in 2.7% of 224 iliac procedures.[2] More recently, Tegtmeyer and co-workers reported on a single-centre series of 200 patients with a technical success of PTA of 88%, a total complication rate of 10.5% and a major complication rate of 6.5%.[3] Follow-up results reported on a 2-year patency of 90% and a 5-year patency of 85% in successfully treated patients. Secondary patency was 99% after 2 years and 92% after 5 years.

It would be difficult to improve on these excellent results. However, the type of lesions treated influences the technical success rate. For example, whether an iliac lesion is eccentric or has a calcified or ulcerated plaque is very significant. Similarly, the occurrence of a dissection or iliac occlusion has a major impact on the technical and probably also the follow-up results. Metallic stenting, therefore, may offer a solution in especially difficult cases, and in patients in whom complications of simple balloon angioplasty have occurred.[1,4]

Stent placement in stenotic lesions is indicated in patients in whom angioplasty has proved inadequate, as defined by visibly poor outflow or major pressure gradients. Since follow-up data are now available showing that iliac stent placement is safe, a liberal approach to problem cases is justified although primary stenting of stenoses is not recommended.

Stenoses

As balloon angioplasty has proved to be an effective procedure especially in the treatment of iliac stenoses, the indication for stent placement should be restricted to lesions which cannot be treated adequately by angioplasty alone. An inadequate post-angioplasty result has been suggested as a general indication for stent placement. Residual pressure gradients are certainly a useful way to assess the success of the procedure, but it is still unclear what is the borderline gradient ultimately requiring additional intervention, and the decision should not be made without reference to both morphological criteria and visibly reduced flow.

Long-segment stenoses with an irregular surface (Fig. 1.2), aneurysm formation or markedly ulcerated plaques (Fig. 1.3) may be included in the group of complex lesions, that may not respond well to angioplasty and should be considered for stent placement. Eccentric stenoses and ostial lesions with extension to the aortic bifurcation are also known not to respond well to balloon angioplasty. Similarly, a stenotic lesion may appear to be adequately dilated by balloon inflation, but may collapse after deflating the balloon.

Complications of balloon angioplasty such as intramural haematoma (Fig. 1.4) are well treatable by stent placement. A flow-obstructing dissection is an indication for immediate stent placement, in order to maintain the vascular lumen and obviate emergency surgery.

Figure 1.2
(a) Eccentric stenosis of left common iliac artery. (b) Full reopening after stenting with use of a Wallstent.

(a)

(b)

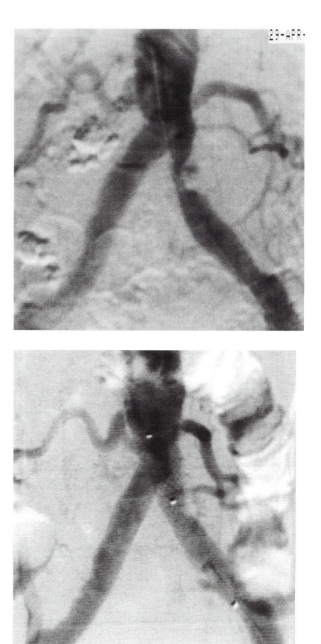

(a)

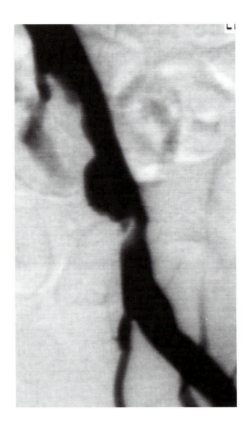

(b)

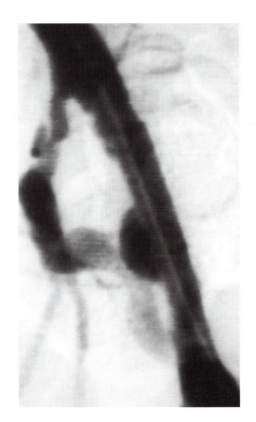

Figure 1.3
(a) Ulcerated plaque within stenosis of left external iliac artery. (b) After stenting the stenosis is gone but the ulceration remains. The ulcer has thrombosed on follow-up examination.

Figure 1.4   (a)
(a) Dissection following angioplasty (arrow). (b) Pseudoaneurysm (arrow) post-angioplasty, becoming symptomatic 1 week after primary PTA.

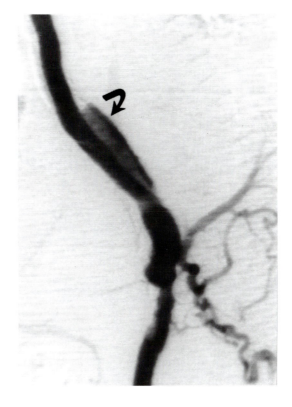

(b)

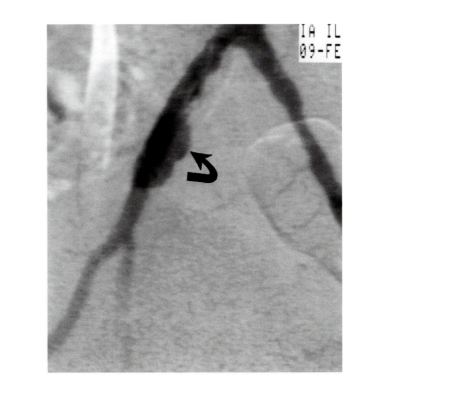

In aortic lesions, the indications for stent placement do not differ considerably from the iliac arteries but some landmarks, such as the ostia of the renal and inferior mesenteric arteries, should be protected. Long-segment Y-shaped stenting of the aortic bifurcation should be used conservatively, because endothelization of the stented segment is unlikely.

In general, iliac restenosis after angioplasty does not require stent placement because in this situation there is no proof that stenting prevents restenosis. However, stenting may be useful when there is an unsatisfactory result from balloon angioplasty.

Occlusions

Metallic stents, especially self-expandable endoprostheses, represent a new concept in percutaneous revascularization of chronic iliac occlusions (Fig. 1.5), which is one of the main indications for stent placement.[4] Self-expandable stents are used to cover the occluding thrombotic material, thereby preventing peripheral dislodgement, a well-known complication of percutaneous treatment of iliac occlusions. Moreover, stent placement maintains the increase of the vascular lumen gained by balloon dilatation, and avoids overdilatation.

Femoral arteries

In femoral arteries the long-term results of balloon angioplasty are less than optimal. Long-segment occlusions and diffuse segmental stenotic disease are known to respond poorly to PTA, with low follow-up patency after 6 months. There is a need to improve both the immediate mid- and long-term results of percutaneous treatment in femoral arteries. However, stent placement has not proved a reliable solution to this problem.

The indications for placement of stents in femoral arteries are, therefore, different from those in iliac arteries. As the frequency of restenosis is high in femoral stents within the first 6 months after placement, their use should be limited to patients with severe flow-impairing dissection, intramural haematoma or other complications of percutaneous balloon angioplasty (Fig. 1.6). Placement could also be considered if PTA is technically unsuccessful in patients with limb-threatening disease, in order to maintain early patency for limb salvage reasons. In any case, the stented segment should be as short as possible.

There are very limited indications for stenting of the common femoral artery, the very proximal superficial femoral and proximal deep femoral artery, as these arteries are easily accessible for surgical treatment.

Stenting of the popliteal segment of the popliteal artery is technically feasible with pliable stents but recurrent flexion of the stent may lead to thrombotic occlusion of the endoprosthesis. This location is also prone to increased neointimal hyperplasia.

Figure 1.5
(a) Chronic occlusion of the left common iliac artery. (b) After inadequate dilatation, endoluminal occlusion material is visible. (c) After stenting, full patency is restored.

(a)

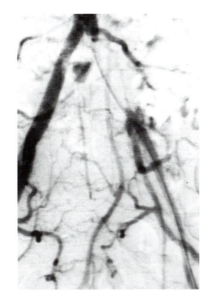

(b)

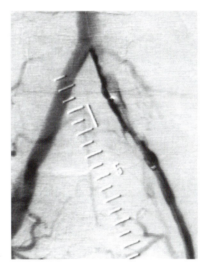

(c)

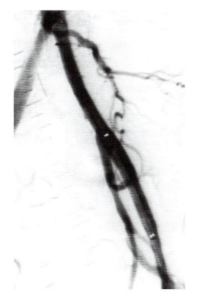

(a)

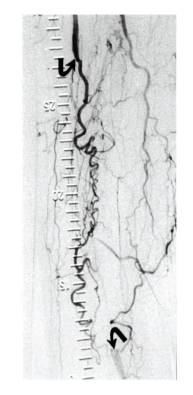

(b)

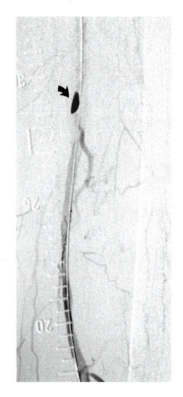

Figure 1.6
(a) Occlusion of left superficial femoral artery (SFA) over 16 cm (arrows). (b) After balloon dilatation, the segment is patent again but a severe dissection remains (arrow) inhibiting full arterial flow. (c) After circumscribed stenting with use of a short Palmaz stent (arrow), the segment is patent.

(c)

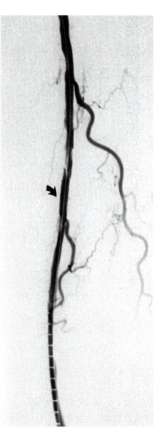

Renal arteries

In the renal arteries, the main indication for stent placement is a technical failure of balloon angioplasty. PTA of the renal arteries is a well-established technique with a low complication rate and high technical success. Clinical success is sometimes difficult to determine. Unfortunately, many patients with essential hypertension may have irrelevant renal artery stenosis which may even be the consequence, rather than the cause, of hypertension.

The restenosis rate in true renal artery stenosis is 20–30%, but is much higher in ostial lesions, which respond poorly to simple PTA (Fig. 1.7).

Figure 1.7
(a) Ostial stenosis of right renal artery. (b) Following PTA, diameter did not much improve. (c) After placement of a Palmaz stent (length 2 cm, diameter 6 mm), the ostium is widely patent.

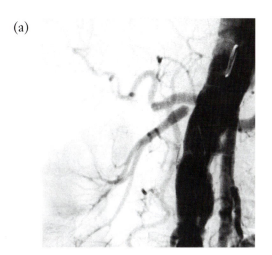

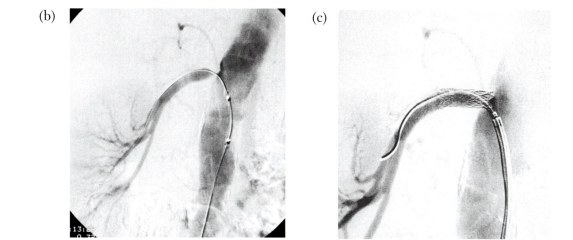

A very conservative approach should be adopted in stenting of the renal arteries. In cases where the morphological result is poor, but flow seems improved, it is the authors' policy to wait and to check haemodynamic improvement by both duplex sonography and clinical outcome. In most cases, primary stenting is limited to severe and flow-impairing dissection. In cases of restenosis, repeat angioplasty may obtain excellent results, and there is no proof that stenting prevents occurrence of this complication.

Possible complications of stenting should be handled with particular care in renal arteries: stent occlusion or restenosis may occur silently with no reliable warning symptoms which allow reintervention in time to preserve function.

Some ostial lesions may benefit from stent placement although results from large series are not yet available. The Palmaz stent is particularly appropriate for renal artery stenting because it can be precisely placed. Placement of the Wallstent can be problematic because antegrade delivery of the stent with stent shortening makes it difficult to position it accurately at the renal ostium; for this reason the Wallstent is not the stent of first choice in the renal arteries.

Visceral arteries

There is very little experience with stenting of visceral arteries such as the coeliac trunk and the superior mesenteric artery. In general, the indication for angioplasty is limited to severe cases with abdominal angina, and stenting may be applied in cases of complicated PTA and dissection.

Supra-aortic arteries

In the subclavian arteries (Fig. 1.8), stent placement may be used secondary to PTA, if balloon angioplasty of a stenosis fails.[5] Primary stenting of subclavian arterial obstructions was performed by Kumar and co-workers who reported excellent technical success.[6]

Primary stenting of carotid arteries followed by PTA is of increasing interest. Stent placement is of theoretical advantage in irregular and ulcerated lesions, allowing a more regular surface appearance after percutaneous treatment. This method might help avoid embolism from the atherosclerotic lesion or angioplasty-induced vascular injury. Stenting could also be helpful to overcome related complications such as dissection.

Clinical results

Aorta and iliac arteries

The indications for stent placement in isolated aortic lesions are relatively rare because of the small number of patients undergoing balloon angioplasty of the aorta, and the good technical results that can be achieved by PTA alone.[7] Bifurcational stenoses may undergo bilateral Y-shaped stenting into the aortic lumen. However, follow-up results are not encouraging and the complication rate is higher than for iliac stent placement.

Wallstent
Iliac stenoses. The authors followed up 118 patients with stented aorto-iliac stenoses.[8] The length of the stenosed segment was 3 ± 2 cm; in 103 patients the

Figure 1.8
(a) Occlusion of left subclavian artery (arrow). (b) After PTA, insufficient and irregular lumen is achieved. (c) After stenting with a Palmaz stent (arrow), follow-up control after 1 year reveals full patency of subclavian artery.

(a)

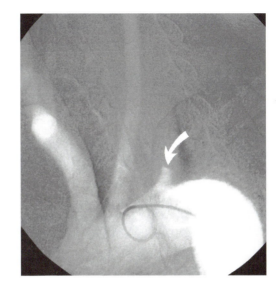

(b)

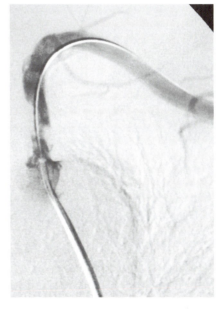

(c)

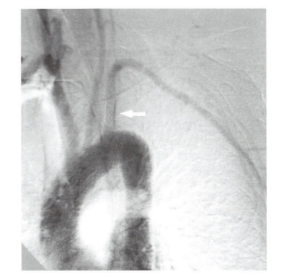

lesion was shorter than 5 cm; in 15 patients it was longer than 5 cm. Morphologically, 85 lesions were eccentric, 73 lesions showed major calcifications and, in 52 lesions, irregular margins were found.

A total of 142 stents was placed with a mean of 1.2 ± 0.5 stents per patient. The mean length of the stented segment was 4 ± 2 cm. The clinical condition improved in 112 patients; 89 patients improved for two more stages. The mean ankle–branchial index significantly improved to 0.92 ± 0.17.

The primary cumulative patency was 97% after 6 months, 95% after 1 year and 88% after 2 years; the 4-year patency was 82%. The secondary or assisted patency was 97% after 6 months, 96% after 1 year and 93% after 2 years. The 3- and 4-year patencies were 91% each.

Chronic iliac occlusions. The authors treated 103 chronic iliac occlusions.[9] The mean length of the occluded segment was 5.1 ± 3.1 cm; in 44 patients the occlusion was shorter than 5 cm (SCVIR class III), in 59 patients it was longer than 5 cm (SCVIR class IV).[9] The lesion included the ostium of the common iliac artery in 48 patients and the ostium of the external iliac artery in 41 patients. The lesion extended into the common femoral artery in 2 patients. The mean ankle–branchial index at rest was 0.48 ± 0.2 prior to treatment.

The average angiographic follow-up period was 26 ± 18 months. The average clinical follow-up period was 29 ± 17 months.

A total of 154 stents was placed with a mean of 1.6 ± 0.7 stents per patient. The mean stented segment was 6.1 ± 3.3 cm. Arterial flow was successfully re-established in 101 patients. In 2 patients, the stent entered the aorta subintimally, thus leading to a compression of the stent entrance. In both patients, further intervention was abandoned and the new channel thrombosed within 24 hours, despite heparinization. Thus, technical success for remodelling the vascular lumen was 98% (101 of 103 patients). The clinical condition improved in 99 patients. The mean ankle–arm index improved to 0.89 ± 0.19.

The primary patency was 92% after 6 months, 87% after 1 year and 83% after 2 years. The 4-year patency was 78%. The secondary or assisted patency was 95% after 6 months, 94% after 1 year and 90% after 2 years. The 3- and 4-year patencies were 88% each.

Complications. The rate of complications in iliac arteries is relatively small. In iliac stenoses, the total complication rate was 6.8% with a major complication rate of 3.4% that included subacute stent thrombosis. In iliac occlusions, complications occurred in 11.7%. An additional surgical or percutaneous reintervention became necessary in 6 patients; thus the major complication rate was 5.8%. The most frequent type of complication in chronic arterial occlusions was arterial emboli.

Reobstruction. In the authors' series, stent reobstruction occurred in 7.6% of stenoses and 17.5% of occlusions. Stent stenoses occurred in 44%, stent occlusions in 56%. Stent stenosis was managed with balloon dilatation and restenting. Stent occlusion was treated by aspiration, atherectomy and additional stent placement (Fig. 1.9).

Palmaz and Strecker stents

For iliac stent placement, larger series with follow-up data are now available for three types of vascular endoprostheses: the Strecker stent, the Palmaz stent and

Figure 1.9
(a) Directional atherectomy within the reoccluded stent in the right external iliac artery. (b) After atherectomy, a smooth lumen is present that can be dilated or restented.

(a)

(b)

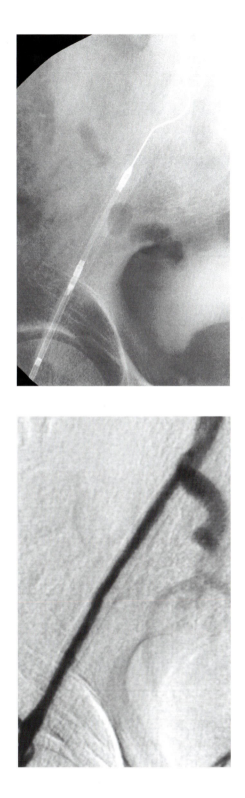

the Wallstent.[10,11] These devices have different patterns of stent design, radial expansile force and surface geometry, which may theoretically influence follow-up results.[12]

A multi-centre study including 486 patients in whom the Palmaz stent was placed revealed a technical success of 99% and a complication rate of 10% with major complications in 4.7%. Clinical follow-up patency was 90% after 1 year and 84% after 2 years.[11]

Strecker and co-workers reported a technical success of 100% in 116 patients with iliac lesions and implantation of a Strecker tantalum stent, and a follow-up patency of 95% at 1 and 2 years each.[10] Recently, Long et al. reported on iliac implantation of Strecker stents in 64 patients. Technical success was 98%, the overall complication rate 12% and the major complication rate 3.1%.[13] They reported restenosis in 10 and reocclusion in 8 cases.

The authors' results with the Wallstent are comparable to those reported in the literature for other types of stents. However, it remains difficult to compare data from different series because several factors such as lesion morphology, the extent of the disease, or outflow conditions, may be different.[9]

There is no obvious difference in technical success and follow-up results for reported different types of metallic stents placed in iliac arteries.

Other stents

At present, few clinical results are available for other types of stent, such as the Cragg non-covered nitinol stent and the low-profile Nitinol Memotherm™ stent (Angiomed, Karlsruhe, Germany). Hausegger et al. reported on their first clinical results with the Cragg stent, with a high technical success.[14] Starck et al. presented follow-up data on 203 patients with the Memotherm stent, reporting a technical success rate of 98%. They used the stent in the iliac (44%) and femoropopliteal (52%) region and reported improved follow-up clinical results when compared with the Strecker stent.[15] These preliminary data, however, remain to be proven by controlled prospective follow-up studies.

Femoral arteries

Wallstent

In femoral arteries, results after placement of the Wallstent are not particularly encouraging. With a mean length of obstruction of 6.6 cm, Sapoval and co-workers[16] had an early stent thrombosis in 4 of 21 cases (19%). Follow-up showed a primary patency of 63% after 6 months and 49% after 1 year. The assisted patency was 72% after 6 months and 67% after 1 year.[16]

The authors' own results were similar. In 25 patients with a mean length of obstruction of 6 cm and a stented segment of 8.5 cm on average, 3 subacute thromboses occurred (12%). Follow-up revealed a primary patency of 83% (6 months) and 55% (12 months) and a secondary patency of 83% (6 months) and 63% (12 months).

Rousseau and co-workers reported better long-term results with a follow-up patency of 76% at 2 years, but also reported a 17% rate of early thrombosis.[17]

Do and co-workers compared stenting with PTA in femoropopliteal occlusions[18] and did not find significant benefits from stenting; they had a 6-month patency of 76% (stents) versus 77% (PTA) and a 1-year patency of 59% (stent) versus 65% (PTA). The average length of occlusion was 8.6 cm (stents) and 6 cm (PTA). The stent thrombosis rate was 19%, while no acute rethrombosis occurred in the PTA group.

These results justify a conservative policy for use of stents in femoral arteries, especially in cases where longer segments of disease have to be covered. The results are more favourable when the stented segment is short; the length of the stented segment seems to be an important factor affecting stent thrombosis and restenosis (Fig. 1.10).

Palmaz and Strecker stents
In femoral arteries, Pinot *et al.* reported a low restenosis rate of 19% in 43 patients treated with Palmaz stents.[19] Henry *et al.* described a primary patency of 72% after 3 years.[20] These results appear better than with Wallstents in the femoral artery. One explanation might be that in most instances the stented segment was kept considerably shorter than in other studies with the Wallstent, where mostly long femoral segments were covered by stents.

The Strecker stent has been used in femoral and popliteal arteries. Strecker *et al.* reported results from a series of 84 femoropopliteal stents.[10] There were 24 cases of reobstruction (29%) and a cumulative patency of 80% after 12 months was calculated. Starck and co-workers[21] produced a life-table analysis on the patency of Strecker stents in femoropopliteal vessels and found a 2-year patency of 52%. These results are comparable to those after placement of the Wallstent.

Figure 1.10
Restenosis within a femoral stent (arrow) due to neointimal hyperplasia 7 months after stent placement.

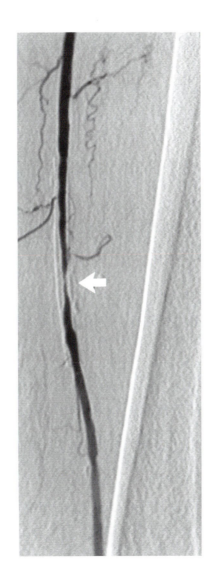

Renal arteries

Wallstent

Joffre et al. have published a series of 17 patients treated with renal arterial stent placement.[22] In all cases, the indication for stenting was incomplete angioplasty. They described technical success in all cases with only 1 case of restenosis. In a more recent paper, the same group reported a restenosis rate of 20% (4 of 21) and a primary patency rate of 95% after 7 months and 77% after 15 months.[23] A series of 18 patients was reported by Raynaud et al.,[24] who found only 1 case of restenosis but had 2 cases with recurrent stenosis or thrombosis out of 10 patients on whom follow-up data were available.[25]

Misplacement of stents has been described by the Toulouse group in 6 of 21 cases with slight but inadvertent protrusion into the aortic lumen in 2 and primary non-covering of ostial lesions in 4 cases. All cases necessitated placement of another stent. In the series by Raynaud et al., in 3 of 18 cases the first stent did not cover the lesion and in 10 out of 18 cases the stent protruded into the aortic lumen up to 5 mm. These data outline the problems of exact placement of the Wallstent in renal arteries. Consequently, Wilms and co-workers[25] inaugurated a modified delivery system of the Wallstent for renal application with a fourth marker for exact placement.

Palmaz and Strecker stents

Rees and co-workers reported on 28 patients with renal artery stenosis treated with placement of a Palmaz stent. There was technical success in 27 out of 28 cases. Of the 18 patients available for follow-up, restenosis occurred in 7 (39%). No stent thrombosis occurred.[26] Dorros and co-workers reported on Palmaz stents placed in 92 stenotic renal arteries. The rate of restenosis was 25%, but 55% of patients with renal insufficiency showed improvement of renal function.[27] Kuhn et al. reported on the use of the Strecker stent for treating renal arterial lesions in 10 patients. Stent misplacement occurred in 3 cases. In 1 case, failure due to stent collapse occurred. Restenosis was reported in 2 of 10 patients.[28]

Thus, the literature of renal artery stenting is limited to small series except for the Dorros paper and there are no significant differences in follow-up results, except for placement problems with both the Wallstent and the Strecker stent.

Supra-aortic arteries

In the subclavian and brachiocephalic arteries, placement of stents helps to reduce the amount of residual stenosis significantly.[5] No significant complications have been reported.[6] Kumar and co-workers[6] used primary stenting with the Palmaz stent to treat subclavian artery obstruction in 31 cases (8 occlusions, 23 stenoses). They encountered one stent dislodgement, but no events of cerebral ischaemia. Recanalization was successful in all cases with a residual stenosis of 6% on average. It is not possible to determine the benefits of primary stenting compared with PTA alone, which renders excellent results in stenoses and occlusions.[5]

Adjunctive medication

In iliac arterial stents, 24-hour medication with intravenous heparin (500–1000 IU/h) and follow-up medication with aspirin (ASA) 100 mg/d seems sufficient. In some cases with reduced in- and outflow, anticoagulation with warfarin for 3 months may be an option. In renal arteries, 3 months of anticoagulation with warfarin is recommended, followed by ASA as a lifetime medication. In femoral arteries, 3 months of anticoagulation or a combination of ticlopidine and ASA for 3 months followed by ASA 100 mg/d is a current regimen.

The combination of ticlopidine and ASA has shown promising results in coronary stenting and may be an option in the early postimplantation phase (3 months) after renal and femoropopliteal stenting.

In cases where stent thrombosis occurs, the authors currently use long-term anticoagulation irrespective of the location of the stent.

Special indications for special stents

Several factors are relevant in choosing one type of stent in preference to another including personal experience, economic resources, length and type of lesions.

In the authors' opinion, the Wallstent has certain advantages in tortuous vessels, chronic occlusions of iliac arteries and long-segment stenoses. In renal arteries, problems with the precision of placement of the Wallstent, especially in ostial lesions, are obvious disadvantages compared with the Palmaz stent. In femoral arteries, short-segment stenting seems important for the achievement of optimal results. Thus, the Palmaz offers advantages over the Wallstent in length reduction and price. However, personal skill, training and experience are very important factors if optimal results are to be achieved.

References

1 Becker G, Katzen B, Dake M. Noncoronary angioplasty. *Radiology* 1989; **170**: 921–940.
2 Gardiner G, Meyerovitz M, Stokes K, Clouse M, Harrington D, Bettmann M. Complications of transluminal angioplasty. *Radiology* 1986; **159**: 201–208.
3 Tegtmeyer C, Hardwell G, Selby B, Robertson R, Kron I, Tribble C. Results and complications of angioplasty in aortoiliac disease. *Circulation* 1991; **83**(Suppl. 2): (I)53–60.
4 Vorwerk D, Guenther RW. Mechanical revascularization of occluded iliac arteries with use of self-expandable endoprostheses. *Radiology* 1990; **175**: 411–415.
5 Mathias K. Perkutane Rekanalisation der supraaortalen und zerebralen Arterien. In: Guenther R W, Thelen M (eds) *Interventionelle Radiologie*. Stuttgart: Thieme, 1996: 112–123.
6 Kumar K, Dorros G, Bates MC, Plamer L, Mathiak L, Dufek C. Primary stent deployment in occlusive subclavian artery disease. *Cathet Cardiovasc Diagn* 1995; **34**: 281–285.
7 Vorwerk D, Guenther RW, Bohndorf K, Keulers P. Stent placement for failed angioplasty of aortic stenoses: report of two cases. *Cardiovasc Intervent Radiol* 1991; **14**: 316–319.
8 Vorwerk D, Guenther RW, Schürmann K, Wendt G. Aortic and iliac stenoses: follow-up results of stent placement after insufficient balloon angioplasty in 118 cases. *Radiology* 1996; **198**: 45–48.
9 Vorwerk D, Guenther RW, Schürmann K, Wendt G, Peters I. Primary stent placement for chronic iliac artery occlusions: follow-up results in 103 patients. *Radiology* 1995; **194**: 745–749.
10 Strecker E, Hagen B, Liermann D, Schneider B, Wolf H, Wambasganss J. Iliac and femoropopliteal vascular occlusive disease treated with flexible tantalum stents. *Cardiovasc Intervent Radiol* 1993; **16**: 158–164.
11 Palmaz JC, Laborde J, Rivera F, Encarnacion C, Lutz J, Moss J. Stenting of the iliac arteries with the Palmaz stent. Experience from a multicenter trial. *Cardiovasc Intervent Radiol* 1992; **15**: 291–297.
12 Schatz R. A view of vascular stents. *Circulation* 1989; **79**: 445–457.
13 Long A, Sapoval M, Beyssen B *et al*. Strecker stent implantation in iliac arteries: patencies and predictive factors for long-term success. *Radiology* 1995; **194**: 739–744.
14 Hausegger KA, Lafer M, Lammer J *et al*. Iliac artery stenting – clinical experience with a nitinol prototype stent (Cragg stent) (abstract). *Cardiovasc Intervent Radiol* 1993; **16**(Suppl.): S25.
15 Starck E, Dukiet C, Heinz C, Vierhauser S. Clinical experience with a new self-expanding nitinol stent (abstract). *Cardiovasc Intervent Radiol* 1995; **18**(Suppl.): S72.
16 Sapoval M, Long A, Raynaud A, Beyssen B, Fiessinger J, Gaux J. Femoropopliteal stent placement: long-term results. *Radiology* 1992; **184**: 833–839.

17 Rousseau H, Raillat C, Joffre F, Knight C, Ginestet M. Treatment of femoropopliteal stenoses by means of self-expandable endoprostheses: mid-term results. *Radiology* 1989; **172**: 961–964.

18 Do DD, Triller J, Walpoth B, Stirnemann P, Mahler F. A comparison study of self-expandable stents vs balloon angioplasty alone in femoropopliteal artery occlusions. *Cardiovasc Intervent Radiol* 1992; **15**: 306–312.

19 Pinot J, Langlois J, Touze J, Bergeron J. SFA Palmaz stent: Long-term results (abstract). *Cardiovasc Intervent Radiol* 1994; **17**(Suppl. 2): S67.

20 Henry M, Amor M, Ethevenot G *et al*. Primary and secondary patency of stented peripheral arteries. Three years follow-up. A single center experience (abstract). *Cardiovasc Intervent Radiol* 1994; **17**(Suppl.): S57.

21 Starck E, Wagner H, Truss J. Erste Life-Table Analyse nach Strecker-Stent-Implantation bei komplizierten Angioplastien. *Vasa Suppl.* 1991; **33**: 199.

22 Joffre F, Rousseau H, Bernadet P *et al*. Midterm results of renal artery stenting. *Cardiovasc Intervent Radiol* 1992; **15**: 313–316.

23 Hennequin L, Joffre F, Rousseau H *et al*. Renal artery stent placement: long-term results with the Wallstent endoprosthesis. *Radiology* 1994; **191**: 713–719.

24 Raynaud A, Beyssen B, Turmel-Rodrigues L *et al*. Renal artery stent placement: immediate and mid-term technical and clinical results. *J Vasc Intervent Radiol* 1994; **5**: 849–858.

25 Wilms G, Peene P, Baert A *et al*. Renal artery stent placement with use of the Wallstent endoprosthesis. *Radiology* 1991; **179**: 457–462.

26 Rees C, Palmaz J, Becker G *et al*. Palmaz stent in atherosclerotic stenoses involving the ostia of the renal arteries: preliminary report of a multicenter study. *Radiology* 1991; **181**: 507–514.

27 Dorros G, Jaff M, Jain A, Dufek C, Mathiak L. Follow-up of primary Palmaz–Schatz stent placement for atherosclerotic renal artery stenosis. *Am J Cardiol* 1995; **75**: 1051–1055.

28 Kuhn F, Kutkuhn B, Torsello G, Mödder U. Renal artery stenosis: preliminary results of treatment with the Strecker stent. *Radiology* 1991; **180**: 367–372.

29 Mathias K, Kempkes U, Jaeger H. Stent placement in complex internal carotid artery lesions (abstract). *Radiology* 1994; **193**: (P) 209.

30 Mathias K, Jaeger H, Mau C, Goetz F. Problems and complications of internal carotid artery percutaneous transluminal angioplasty and stent placement (abstract). *Radiology* 1995; **197**: (P) 234.

31 Theron J. Present experience in endovascular treatment of atherosclerotic stenoses of the carotid bifurcation (abstract). *Radiology* 1995; **197**: (P) 205.

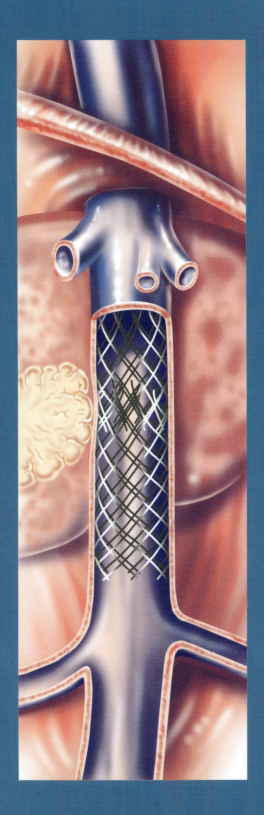

Chapter 2
Metal stents in the venous system

R.F. Dondelinger, P. Capasso, T. Tancredi and G. Trotteur

Introduction

Venous obstruction has not attracted as much attention as arterial flow impairment from interventional radiologists. However, occlusion of large veins is not a rare event and can be responsible for dramatic symptoms and occasionally even be lethal. The potential of the venous system to collateralize, and the usually non-lethal nature of venous obstruction, are the two main reasons why, in most cases, conservative medical management is applied to occlusion of peripheral or large central veins.

In contrast to its application in arterial stenoses, percutaneous transluminal angioplasty (PTA) is only occasionally successful in veins. In the initial reports, which date back to the late 1970s and 1980s, a high restenosis rate was observed.[1–6] The main mechanisms of reocclusion are elastic recoil of the venous wall, mural fibrosis, intimal hyperplasia, persistent perivascular compression by tumour, and endoluminal tumour growth. Conditions leading to poor flow or to injury to the venous endothelium or valves can also lead to rapid rethrombosis. Repeated dilatations with high-pressure balloons, laser-assisted PTA, or simultaneous inflation of several balloons placed side by side in the caval veins have not been consistently successful.[7–9] The rationale for using expandable metal stents is the immediate and permanent achievement of venous patency, obviating more invasive surgery.[10]

Animal experiments

Only a small number of experimental studies were conducted in animal models prior to the clinical application of metal stents in venous obstruction in humans. These studies proved both the biocompatibility and the efficacy of the stents. In earlier attempts, a spiral metal stent designed by Maas was placed in the inferior vena cava (IVC) of dogs and calves through a venotomy.[11] The stents remained patent, without side effects, for as long as 2 years; however, the Maas stent was not used clinically. Gianturco™ Z-stents (William Cook Europe, A/S Bjaeverskov, Denmark) were tested more extensively in various models. A stenosis of the IVC in dogs was created by pericaval injection of absolute ethanol, resulting in at least a 50% local reduction of luminal diameter and a transstenotic pressure gradient of $5\,cmH_2O$. Stents that were placed percutaneously within the stenosis remained open for several months without adjuvant anticoagulation or anti-platelet medication. The stents were largely and rapidly incorporated in the caval wall. When barbs were added to the stents, no displacement was noticed.[12] Palmaz® stents (Johnson & Johnson,

Warren, NJ, USA) were experimentally evaluated in the venous system, mainly in tributaries of the caval system, owing to the initially limited diameter of the stent. Complete neo-endothelial covering of the stents and mid-term venous patency was confirmed, but migration occurred.[13] Other experiments using pigs have shown a decreased deposit of indium-labelled platelets in iliac veins after stenting of a 4-week-old stricture created by catgut ligation. Interestingly, arterial stents used in the same animal model showed increased thrombogenicity.[14] Tantalum wire stents were used in medium-size veins of dogs. Patency of stented veins and sidebranches was documented, with a low morbidity in terms of stent migration and deformation.[15] Stents were also placed in anastomotic stenoses of reversed vein grafts in sheep. Neointimal coverage and maintenance of graft patency was demonstrated. The major cause of stent occlusion in this study was incomplete stent–vessel wall contact.[16]

Clinical indications

Potential indications for percutaneous stenting are stenoses of the superior vena cava (SVC), the innominate veins,[17–27] the IVC and iliofemoral veins,[19,21–3,25,26,28–30] mainly caused by primary or secondary malignant tumours. Stenoses of benign origin include stenosed haemodialysis shunts,[31–7] postoperative or graft anastomotic stenoses in the caval or portal system,[38–41] Budd–Chiari syndrome,[42–50] iliac vein compression or May–Turner syndrome,[51] and post-thrombotic occlusion.[52–8]

Superior vena caval obstruction

Clinical symptoms
Vena caval obstruction causes marked distress and anxiety. The SVC syndrome can develop progressively or acutely. Clinical symptoms include headache, which is exacerbated during changes of position, disturbances of consciousness, oedema, tension or pain in the face and neck, blurred vision, retro-orbital pressure, and orthopnoea. Oedema and pain can involve one or both arms. Collateral circulation develops to a variable degree over the chest wall and periscapular region.

Malignant obstruction
Most strictures of the caval system and venous tributaries are of malignant origin. Development of the SVC syndrome may be the first sign of a mediastinal tumour, or may be seen later in the course of the disease, and even occur after surgery, radiotherapy or chemotherapy.[17] The tumours most commonly responsible for compression of the SVC and large mediastinal veins are bronchogenic carcinoma or small-cell lung cancer with mediastinal lymph node enlargement caused by metastases from intra- or extrathoracic malignancies, malignant lymphoma or Hodgkin's disease, and tracheal malignancies. Other primary mediastinal tumours are less often encountered. The traditional method of treatment of SVC obstruction due to malignancy is radiotherapy or chemotherapy, or a combination of both. This is effective in about 90% of cases, but only after several days, and with a recurrence rate of 20%, even when the maximum permissible dose of radiation is used.[17,59] High-grade SVC obstruction unresponsive to treatment may lead to thrombosis.[18] Therefore, patients with involvement of the confluence

of the innominate veins should be treated early, even if not fully symptomatic, as percutaneous reconstruction of the caval bifurcation with stents becomes more hazardous when a Y-shaped stricture has occurred, requiring multiple, bilateral stents. Although in the first reports patients were considered for endoluminal stenting only after an initial attempt of radio- or chemotherapy, the high success rate and minimal morbidity associated with the procedure has led to its use as a first choice, even in patients with a short life expectancy.[22,27,59] Stenting of the caval system or other large mediastinal veins produces rapid and marked improvement of the quality of life, secondary to the disappearance of congestive symptoms. An SVC pressure higher than 22 mmHg is usually present above the obstruction in symptomatic patients.[24]

In patients given nephrotoxic chemotherapy, such as cisplatin, cyclophosphamide, isosfamide, methotrexate, bleomycin, streptozotocin, pentostatin, or other nephrotoxic drugs, and in patients in whom extensive tumour lysis with hyperuricaemia and hypercalcaemia and emesis-related dehydration is expected during chemotherapy, high-volume hydration – as much as 3 litres of fluid per day – is required. Vena caval stenosis should be treated before chemotherapy is initiated in these patients, to facilitate venous return, even in the presence of minimal symptoms of SVC obstruction.[23]

Inferior vena caval obstruction

Obstruction of the IVC causes venous claudication, and oedema of the lower limbs, pelvis, perineum, scrotum and the abdominal wall. Renal dysfunction may develop. When the hepatic veins are obstructed, hepatocellular function is altered, and hepatomegaly and ascites may ensue. IVC or iliac vein stenoses do not usually lead to severe clinical symptoms necessitating stent placement. Obstruction of malignant origin may be attributable to compression of the IVC by hepatic tumour, or retroperitoneal metastatic lymph node enlargement caused by pelvic malignancies, such as prostatic, cervical, ovarian, bladder and other carcinomas.[28]

Contraindications

In malignant disease, contraindications to venous stenting include extensive thrombosis, anatomical considerations predisposing to severe technical difficulties, and advanced disease in preterminal patients. As a rule, venous accesses should be preserved and the ostia of large tributaries of the caval system, such as the renal, hepatic, innominate, jugular or internal iliac veins, should not be deliberately occluded by a stent, preserving the possibility of further catheterization, if necessary. However, the ostium of the azygos vein is routinely occluded when stenting the SVC, generally without clinical side effects, even when covered stents are used. Impaired venous flow due to limb paralysis is a relative contraindication to stent placement in the iliac or innominate vein. Occasionally, transmural venous tumour invasion is present, caused by lymphoma or bronchogenic carcinoma. Uncovered-stent placement may be ineffective in such cases, and placement of Dacron or other polymer-coated stents is indicated (Fig. 2.1).

Patients should be able to cooperate during the procedure. Some patients with severely symptomatic SVC syndrome may have difficulty in lying flat. In these

(a)

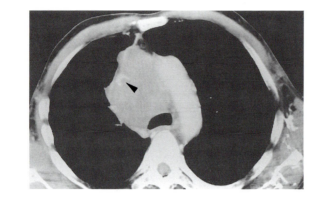

(b)

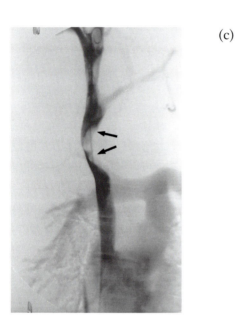

(c)

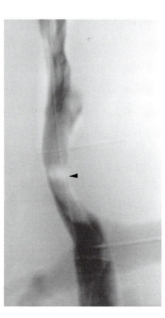

(d)

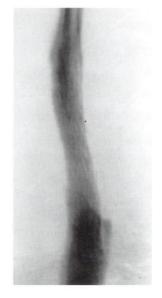

Figure 2.1
55-year-old male, presenting with an SVC syndrome. (a) CT shows a large mediastinal mass compressing or invading the SVC (arrowhead). Histology confirmed malignant non-Hodgkin lymphoma. (b) Superior vena cavography confirms a flattening of the SVC by external compression or invasion (arrows). (c) A Cragg-EndoPro (MinTec, Freeport, Grand Bahama) covered stent was placed (diameter: 12 mm; length: 3 cm) in the SVC by a right femoral approach. Phlebography shows a heterogeneous lumen of the stent (arrowhead), probably caused by partial stent expansion. (d) Following PTA with a 12 mm balloon, optimal flow is achieved.

circumstances, the procedure should be undertaken under general anaesthesia. A minority of patients will present with simultaneous tracheobronchial narrowing due to malignant compression. Stenting of the airways should precede management of the caval obstruction in such patients.

Stenting of benign venous stenoses is undertaken less frequently than in cancer patients. Relative contraindications are discussed below.

Stenting technique

Radiographic technique

Caval obstruction is suggested by the observation of the above-mentioned clinical signs. Duplex and colour-coded Doppler demonstrate stenoses and confirm thrombosis of venous segments accessible to the probe. In most cases, spiral CT with multiplanar reformatting and magnetic resonance angiography can establish an unequivocal diagnosis of central venous stenosis or obstruction; both modalities demonstrate the location and extent of the disease, and also show the collateral network. However, phlebographic demonstration of the stenosis and collateral pathways remains mandatory prior to treatment. Phlebography confirms the location, number and extent of the stenoses, the segmental or web-like shape, thrombi or endoluminal tumour proliferation, extent of collateral circulation, the haemodynamic significance, and any congenital variants to be taken into consideration when planning stent placement. Biplanar superior or inferior cavograms are routinely obtained. Superior venacavography is performed by simultaneous bilateral injection of 25 ml of a non-ionic contrast medium into the basilic or axillary veins, or other more peripheral veins in the upper limb. Inferior venacavography is performed by bilateral femoral vein injection. When puncture of the axillary or femoral vein is problematic due to oedema, CO_2 phlebography may be obtained by a peripheral automatic or hand injection of 60 ml CO_2 into a more proximal venous trunk.

Management of venous thrombosis

When venous thrombosis masks the lesion, local thrombolysis or mechanical thrombectomy should precede stent placement.[22,23,28,39,41,51,52,60] Local thrombolytic infusion seems to give superior results to systemic infusion. A plasminogen activator is infused through an arm vein or by an axillary vein puncture for the SVC and via a femoral approach for the IVC. In some cases of bilateral iliac vein or IVC thrombosis, a jugular vein approach is more convenient. The authors usually place a 5 Fr haemostatic valve sheath at the puncture site. A 3 Fr or 5 Fr catheter with multiple sideholes, or an injectable guidewire, is embedded in the caudal segment of the thrombus and infusion is started. When bilateral iliac or innominate vein thrombosis is present, simultaneous bilateral infusion is used. When complete iliocaval thrombosis is present, the authors do not place a temporary caval filter routinely; however, this may be helpful in selected cases, as systemic thrombolysis of iliac vein thrombosis is associated with pulmonary embolism in up to 6% of cases.[61] Thrombosis of the IVC and SVC does not usually pose an immediate threat to life. Therefore, the authors advocate progressive thrombolysis rather than mechanical thrombectomy, which may be associated with a higher incidence of complications (Fig. 2.2). The authors use urokinase as a plasminogen activator, at an infusion rate

(a)

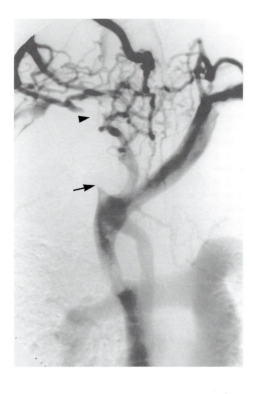

(b)

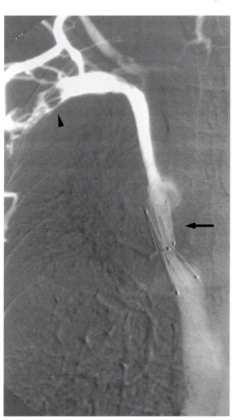

Figure 2.2
66-year-old male, treated for mediastinal small-cell lung cancer, presented with a superior vena cava syndrome. (a) Superior vena cavography showed complete obstruction of the right innominate vein (arrow) and stenosis of the SVC. (b) Following local thrombolysis using urokinase infusion, a 10 mm Wallstent™ (Schneider, AG, Bulach, Switzerland) endoprosthesis was placed in the right innominate vein and a 2 cm double Gianturco stent in the SVC. Phlebography performed immediately after stenting shows restoration of flow and partial expansion of the Z-stent (arrow) and Wallstent endoprosthesis. A small persistent thrombus is seen in the right subclavian vein (arrowhead).

of 75,000 to 100,000 IU/h administered via an automatic pump. Urokinase infusion at moderate dose regimens is associated with few side effects, in the authors' experience, provided cognizance is taken of the generally accepted major contraindications. In particular, patients with episodes of haemoptysis due to bronchogenic carcinoma should not receive thrombolysis.

The entire length of the thrombus is traversed with a guidewire to detect an underlying stenosis. Any stenosis or occlusion that can be traversed with a guidewire can eventually be lysed; therefore, limiting attempts at thrombolysis to such lesions minimizes the technical failure. The thrombus is infiltrated with an average dose of 225,000 IU urokinase before starting infusion. The ease with which the guidewire crosses the obstruction is a good predictor of a successful outcome. Percutaneous thrombus aspiration has been used, either alone or in combination with local thrombolysis; however, technical considerations related to the small diameter of catheters and other devices available render thrombus aspiration alone ineffective in large veins. Other mechanical devices, such as the Amplatz clot macerator, the hydrolyser catheter and others, have been used to clear veins from thrombus. Most of these devices are suitable for smaller veins and do not function optimally in the caval system. Check phlebography is carried out 12–24 hours after the start of plasminogen activator infusion. If this shows that no progress has been achieved, despite correct catheter placement and adequate infusion, the venous segment is probed again with the guidewire to detect any underlying stenosis.

Occasionally, angioplasty is carried out to fragment the clots and expose a greater surface to the plasminogen activator, thus accelerating the thrombolytic process. More recently, a PTA balloon with micropores has been proposed, filled with a thrombolytic agent that is released during inflation; however, migration of thrombi appears to be a frequent event.[60] If partial lysis is achieved, the infusion catheter is placed further distally in the thrombus. During catheterization of obstructed arm veins, care is taken to infuse the basilic vein, and to avoid catheterization and lysis into a smaller collateral branch, as this delays the thrombolytic process. Patients undergoing local venous thrombolytic infusion are not routinely placed in the intensive care unit, as there is no need for the limb to be scrutinized for critical ischaemia. When control phlebography evidences a stenosis, percutaneous stenting is performed immediately to ensure flow. If there are residual thrombi following placement of the stent, thrombolytic infusion is continued. In large veins, local thrombolysis is usually continued for 1–3 days. Complications at the puncture site are rare compared with local arterial infusion, for equivalent doses and an equivalent duration of therapy. Pericatheter thrombosis may be observed in poor flow conditions, but pulmonary embolism is usually not a clinical concern.

Low-dose anticoagulant therapy is sometimes given concurrently with local thrombolysis, mainly when the haemostatic valve sheath is placed in small arm veins, with a reduced flow. The authors infuse 300 U/h heparin continuously through the haemostatic valve sheath to keep the infusion catheter free of thrombi. Coagulation parameters are checked 3 or 4 times per day.

Choice of the venous approach

Stenoses located in the SVC or right innominate vein are best stented via a right femoral approach (Fig. 2.3). Stenoses of the left innominate vein are treated either via a femoral or a left axillary approach. Using a rather unconventional

(a)

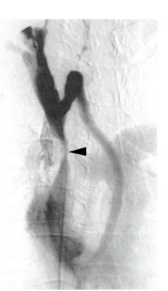

(b)

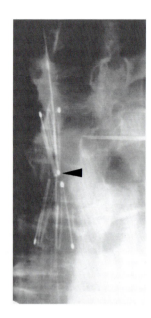

(c)

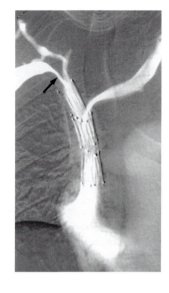

(d)

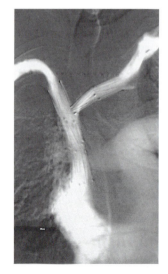

(e)

Figure 2.3
83-year-old male with recurrent bronchogenic adenocarcinoma. A superior vena cava syndrome was treated by radiotherapy 8 months before. Clinical symptoms recurred. (a) Superior vena cavography shows a tight stenosis (arrowhead) of the SVC. (b) A double Z-stent, 2 cm in diameter, was placed in the SVC. The limbs of the cranial stent remained clustered in the stenosis (arrowhead). (c) An additional set of stents was placed and PTA was performed using a 10 mm balloon. (d) Phlebography performed immediately after stenting shows a stenosis of the right subclavian vein (arrow), not covered by the stents, and also narrowing of the left innominate vein. (e) The stenosis of the right subclavian vein was treated with a 10 mm Wallstent endoprosthesis. A double Z-stent was placed in the left innominate vein by an axillary approach. Phlebography confirms optimal flow.

puncture site for catheterization of the axillary vein, at the junction between the axillary and subclavian veins, trauma to the brachial nervous plexus is avoided, particularly when large-diameter catheters are introduced. A more direct access to the left innominate vein is also gained by use of this technique. As a general rule, venous stents should be placed sequentially, first in a distal position then more proximally, in relation to the puncture site. When the confluence of the innominate veins is treated, the technique used depends on the anatomy and the type of stents required. Wallstent™ (Schneider) endoprostheses can be placed simultaneously in the brachiocephalic vein and the left innominate vein, with a parallel course in the SVC. When more rigid stents are used, the SVC and right innominate vein are stented in a line, and stents are placed in the left innominate vein as close as possible to the caval axis. Transoesophageal ultrasound can occasionally be helpful in accurate stent placement in the SVC.[62,63]

All guidewires and catheters must be withdrawn from the segment to be stented before release of the stents, except the guidewire contained in the delivery catheter. In the authors' experience, recanalization of tight occlusions of the left innominate vein, as may be caused by mediastinal tumour or fibrosis, sometimes requires a combined femoral and axillary or a bilateral axillary approach. When the guidewire has crossed the occlusion, it is grasped with a snare, a basket or a flexible forceps on the other side, and retrieved through the haemostatic valve sheath at the second percutaneous entry point. This makes it possible to insert a PTA catheter or any other introducer catheter over the guidewire, which is controlled and straightened at both ends.

The right femoral vein provides the most direct route for stenting the IVC (Fig. 2.4). As the left iliac vein has a more tortuous course, the introduction of a large-calibre delivery catheter may prove difficult, and perforation is a risk. Advancing long and rigid metal stents through an introducer in the left iliac vein may also be difficult (Fig. 2.5). Perforation of the thin wall of the introducer catheter by the metal stents has been observed. The tortuous course may also prevent a correctly centred stent placement and deployment in the caudal IVC. Iliac stents are usually inserted via an ipsilateral femoral approach. Use of the iliac crossover technique is not recommended when rigid stents or large-calibre introducer systems are necessary. When stents have to be placed in the femoral vein, an ipsilateral popliteal approach may be useful with the patient prone. The popliteal vein can be localized by Doppler or by a peripheral injection of iodinated contrast medium or CO_2. Transfixation of both the popliteal artery and vein should be avoided, as it might be complicated by an arteriovenous fistula, which can be treated by external compression with colour-coded Doppler guidance.

The hepatic veins are stented before the IVC. In exceptional circumstances, a transhepatic approach can be used to stent a hepatic vein stenosis.

Adjuvant medication

In apprehensive patients, premedication may be helpful. As endovascular stent placement is not painful, only local anaesthesia at the puncture site is required. PTA is occasionally painful, when the adventitia is stretched during full dilatation. Dilatation of stenoses of peripheral haemodialysis fistulae may also be painful; local infiltration with anaesthetics can be helpful. Patients may also experience pain briefly, following sudden expansion of a metal stent in the

(a)

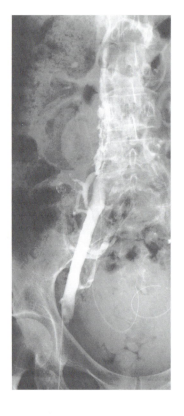

(b)

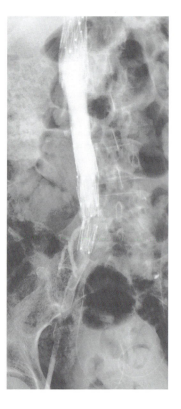

(c)

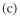

Figure 2.4
54-year-old female with advanced carcinoma of the cervix. Extensive phlebothrombosis of the left lower limb was present and the patient also complained of severe swelling of the right leg. CT evidenced pelvic and retroperitoneal metastatic adenopathies. (a) Right femoral phlebography shows a patent iliac vein and obstruction of the IVC. (b) One set of two Z-stents and another set of three Z-stents (diameter: 2 cm; length: 5 cm) were placed in the caudal IVC. Two additional double stents (diameter: 3.5 cm; length: 5 cm) were placed in the suprarenal IVC. (c) Optimal flow was obtained. The patient became free of symptoms until death 3 months after stenting. Autopsy showed almost complete covering of the stent by a neoendothelium, without narrowing of the caval lumen.

Figure 2.5
79-year-old male, presenting with prostatic carcinoma and bilateral iliac metastatic adenopathies. (a) Bilateral lower limb phlebography shows compression of the common iliac veins, predominating on the left side (arrows). (b) Five double Z-stents (diameter: 2 cm; length: 5 cm) were placed in both iliac veins and the IVC, by a bilateral femoral approach. Improvement of flow was documented immediately after stenting. (c) A radiograph taken 5 days after stenting shows full dilatation of the stents. Pressure in the infrarenal IVC was 15 cmH₂O and central venous pressure 13 cmH₂O. The patient was not significantly improved.

(a)

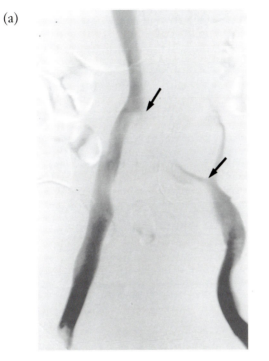

(b)

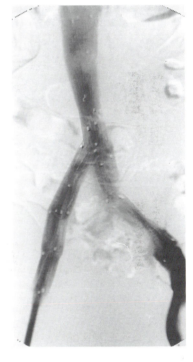

(c)

superior vena cava, and should be warned of this possibility. If it is anticipated that the stenting procedure will be difficult and prolonged, 5000 IU heparin should be given to prevent acute SVC thrombosis, which can be lethal. If SVC stent placement results in immediate and full restoration of flow there is no need for post-stenting heparinization. However, if residual thrombi remain adherent to the stent or vessel wall after local thrombolysis, or if only suboptimal flow has been achieved, full heparinization is given for several days. A partial thromboplastin time of 1.5 to 2.0 times normal should be maintained. Heparinization is followed by oral anticoagulant therapy and low-dose aspirin for several months, by which time it is anticipated that the stent will be completely covered with a neo-endothelium; however, the benefit of this treatment has not been proven. In some patients, stent placement may result in overload due to reperfusion, leading to increased right atrial pressure and transient cardiac decompensation. In patients at risk, pressure monitoring is mandatory during stent placement.[24]

If stent thrombosis occurs rapidly after placement, local infusion of a thrombolytic agent can be performed, as described above. The cause of reocclusion must be determined and treated as appropriate. This may include placement of additional stents, redilatation, or treatment of another stenosis, the significance of which had been previously underestimated.

Type of stents used

All types of metal stents available, either balloon-expandable or self-expanding, can be placed in the venous system. However, treatment of stenoses in large veins requires the use of stents of sufficiently large calibre.

Gianturco or Z-type stents

Gianturco or Z-stents are self-expanding, and available in a double or multiple stent configuration, each segment measuring 2.5 cm in length. They are suitable for use in the SVC, the IVC or other large veins, as they are available in diameters up to 4 cm, which is particularly useful for lesions in the retrohepatic IVC.[19,22–4,30] Distal migration is prevented by small protruding hooks or barbs, which anchor the stent in the vascular wall. Barbs are mandatory, pointing in the two opposite directions to ensure optimal stent stability.[21,22,27] Modifications of the original Gianturco stent include the Rösch-type stent, which incorporates a monofilament to limit expansion or has a spiral configuration to increase flexibility.[17,18,20] Furui has used modified long segmental Z-stents with a variable diameter conforming to that of the venae cavae.[19,30] The introducer sheaths for the larger stents have a diameter of 12–14 Fr. During a long procedure, the lumen of the delivery catheter may occlude rapidly because of accumulation of a considerable volume of clots. In order to prevent this, continuous flushing of the catheter with saline is mandatory. The stent introducers may kink easily, and venous curves are sometimes difficult to negotiate. Z-stents are supplied in a collapsed state in a loading cartridge. When not correctly loaded in the delivery catheter, the partially protruding barbs may lacerate the catheter wall during introduction. Single Gianturco stents should not be used for primary placement, as their placement is difficult to control and they regularly slip beyond the stenosis, or remain in an unstable position within the stenosis and are easily displaced when the stent is recatheterized with a guidewire or a catheter. It is, therefore, advisable to use at least 2-segment Z-stents.[22,23,27,30] However, even double stents are sometimes difficult to centre within the stenosis and they have the tendency to sit on each side of the narrowing, leaving the stenosis uncovered by the metal.

When 3-segment stents are used, the middle stent is placed within the stricture, the two other segments functioning as an anchoring system. A complementary single stent or a double stent can be placed within a multisegment stent already in place to achieve full expansion by placement in an overlapping position. The diameter of the Z-stent is chosen in such a way that the fully expanded stent is 1.2 to 1.5 times the venous diameter. When a double stent is used in a tight stenosis, it may happen that the segment lying within the stricture remains cone-shaped. The struts of the stent remain clustered together in the stenotic channel and lead to thrombosis. Catheterization with a guidewire may then become difficult or impossible. Guidewires with a straight tip should not be used within Z-stents, as they may pass easily between the stent and the venous wall; J-shaped guidewires with a large curve are preferred for that reason. When introducing an angioplasty balloon, the stent may be displaced distally by the balloon catheter, despite resistance from the anchoring barbs. In order to avoid stent displacement, only low-profile balloons should be used to accelerate stent expansion. Balloon expansion of the stent prevents local thrombosis, and rearranges the struts of the stent in a parallel position. When double stents are placed around a curve, the stents may assume an eccentric position. In each case, confirmation of the guidewire position inside the lumen of the already inserted stent must be ascertained before adding an overlapping stent. The stents are very radio-opaque and are clearly visualized during fluoroscopic monitoring of deployment.

Once a Gianturco stent has been extruded from the introducer sheath, relocation is almost impossible. The distal end of a double set of Z-stents may protrude from the left innominate vein into the SVC or from the SVC or IVC into the right atrium, usually without causing complications or cardiac arrythmias. When expanded in the SVC or IVC, Z-stents show an elliptical configuration with a larger anteroposterior than frontal diameter. This is due to the fact that stent expansion is limited in the SVC by the mediastinal pleura and the endothoracic fascia laterally and medially by the adventitia of the ascending thoracic aorta.

Wallstent endoprostheses
Wallstent endoprostheses, with a diameter of 16, 20 and 21 mm, are suitable for stenting of large mediastinal veins, the SVC and IVC , the portal vein and haemodialysis shunt stenoses[26,29,32,34,39] (Fig. 2.6). They require a 9 Fr or a 11.5 Fr introducer sheath. Large Wallstent endoprostheses exhibit an acceptable radio-opacity during fluoroscopic monitoring. Stents loaded within introducer systems that do not utilize a rolling membrane can be retracted again inside the catheter and repositioned even after partial release. Shortening of the stent during expansion is unpredictable in venous stenoses. It should be remembered that the stent shortens considerably when it is allowed to reach full expansion. Wallstent endoprostheses are constrained within a flexible introducer catheter, allowing easy negotiation of venous curves, particularly in tortuous veins. Wallstent endoprostheses are more easily centred in strictures than Gianturco stents. Coaxial placement of several Wallstent endoprostheses is often necessary

(a)
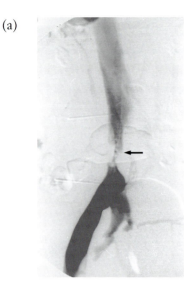

(b)
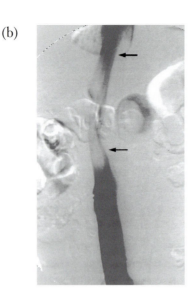

(c)
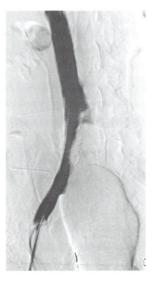

(d)
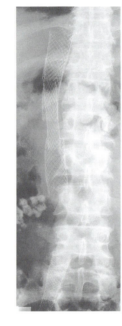

(e)
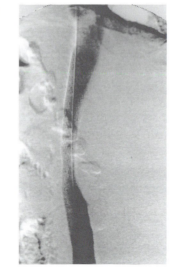

(f)

Figure 2.6

74-year-old male with prostatic carcinoma and retroperitoneal metastatic adenopathies, causing oedema of the legs. (a) Inferior cavography performed via the right femoral vein shows an irregular stenosis (arrow) in the caudal IVC caused by external compression. (b), (c) The suprarenal IVC is also severely compressed (arrows) by retroperitoneal adenopathies, as shown in a frontal and sagittal projection. (d) Four Wallstent endoprostheses with a diameter of 16 mm were placed in the right common iliac vein and the IVC. (e), (f) Optimal flow was achieved in the IVC. The patient improved significantly after stenting.

because of the limited length of these devices. A deployed stent may be easily displaced, as no anchoring hooks are present and veins are very elastic.

Palmaz stents
Palmaz stents have been used in the treatment of haemodialysis stenoses and stenoses in the SVC, IVC, hepatic veins, and other veins in adults and in children.[25,28,38,54,62,64]

Results

Malignant stenoses

In patients with malignant SVC or IVC obstruction, cure of the primary condition is rare. Furthermore, as the life expectancy of patients with irresectable mediastinal or abdominal tumour is limited, the main aim of treatment should be immediate relief from disabling symptoms. PTA alone is rarely effective and should not be considered in such patients. The long-term effects of stent placement are not a major concern. Following successful stent deployment, almost immediate complete or partial relief from symptoms is obtained in 68–100% of cases, at follow-up of up to 16 months, without any need for further intervention.[19–22,26–8,65] In the authors' own experience, 85% of patients remained symptom free after stenting until death.[23] The best results are obtained in the SVC, IVC, innominate and iliac veins. Results tend to be less favourable when circumferential tumour encasement is shown by CT.[19] Successful results are less frequently obtained when stents are placed in more peripheral veins, such as the subclavian or femoral. Patients experience relief of tension in the face and neck almost immediately after stent expansion in the SVC, and the remaining symptoms disappear within a few hours. Oedema of the face and neck resolves after 1–2 days, and in the scapular region and upper limbs in 2–3 days. Although the radial force of metal stents is moderate, they expand almost completely within a week.

No significant difference has been demonstrated in the clinical results following placement of different types of stent. In one report, stent reocclusion was observed in 14%.[21] The left innominate vein is particularly prone to tumour encasement because of its long transverse course through the mediastinum. This vein and the SVC are the veins most frequently infiltrated by tumour, leading to reobstruction. Also, the junction of the left innominate vein and SVC can present an obstacle to stenting. Stent placement should be considered at the onset of clinical symptoms, before a tight stenosis or occlusion involving the SVC bifurcation occurs. Although it may not be necessary to stent both innominate veins to achieve a good clinical result, bilateral stenting helps to re-establish optimal flow and limit the number of reinterventions. Relief of IVC obstruction achieves similar results to SVC stenting, but complete resolution of symptoms may take several weeks or even months.[23,28,30] The clinical benefit gained from caval stenting does not seem to be related to the severity or the duration of obstruction.

Treatment of stent occlusion includes local thrombolysis, thrombectomy, balloon dilatation and placement of additional stents. The possible causes of occlusion are intraluminal tumour growth, progressive tumour growth at the free ends of the stent due to insufficient coverage of the strictures by the stent, vessel contraction, or an inadequate stent diameter leading to central migration. Neointimal proliferation inside the stent usually causes only limited reduction in the caval diameter, and does not usually lead to significant caval restenosis or thrombosis. When obstruction of a stent occurs and is unresponsive to local thrombolysis, the likely cause is tumour infiltration; the diagnosis can be established by endovascular biopsy, using a directional atherectomy catheter.

Benign stenoses

Indications

Approximately 3% of all clinically significant SVC stenoses are due to a benign cause. The main causes of benign stenoses are catheter-related injury, haemodialysis shunt-related obstruction, mediastinal fibrosis secondary to trauma, surgery, post-anastomotic stenoses, infection, radiotherapy, Budd–Chiari syndrome and other rare causes of external compression, such as Ormond disease or polycystic liver. Repeated angioplasty is usually unsuccessful in benign lesions. Traditional treatment of benign obstruction of large veins includes operative veno-venous bypasses or prosthetic grafting, which may expose the patient to the risk of late anastomotic stenosis or graft retraction. A surgically bypassable benign stenosis, occurring in a young symptomatic patient, is a contraindication to stenting, as the long-term behaviour of metal stents in the vascular system is not yet known. An asymptomatic benign lesion should not be stented.

Benign stenoses should always be probed with a balloon, to prove distensibility of the venous wall before stent placement. PTA before stenting is helpful, as the inflated balloon localizes the stenosis precisely; the location of the waist of the balloon can be marked with a radio-opaque marker. Benign stenoses are usually more resistant than malignant strictures. Stenoses that resist to PTA should not be stented, as partial opening of a stent in a high-grade stenosis may precipitate thrombosis. Heparinization and meticulous attention to details of technique are particularly important in such patients.

Budd–Chiari and pseudo-Budd–Chiari syndrome

Budd–Chiari syndrome (BCS) is caused by thrombosis, long segmental stenosis, or membranous webs of the hepatic veins and/or the distal inferior vena cava. In Western countries, BCS is usually caused by extensive thrombosis of the hepatic venous outflow, whereas most cases of membranous webs are reported in patients from the Far East. PTA was unsuccessful in 50% of patients reported in the literature after a 6-month follow-up.[66] When PTA is successful, repeated dilatations may be necessary to maintain patency. Reocclusion of a long segmental stenosis of the IVC at one year is almost invariable, despite prolonged anticoagulation and repeated dilatation. BCS caused by diffuse thrombosis and accompanied by impairment of liver function is treated with portocaval shunting, transjugular intrahepatic portosystemic shunt (TIPS), or liver transplantation. Membranous obstruction or long segmental stenosis of the hepatic veins or the retrohepatic IVC can be corrected by metal stents (Fig. 2.7). Only a few series of patients with BCS treated with metal stents have been reported in the literature;[42,47] most published papers are case reports or reports of short series of patients.[43–6,48–50]

Either the IVC or hepatic veins or both are stented. Intrahepatic venous connections allow decompression of venous outflow following restoration of flow

Figure 2.7
46-year-old male with progressive liver insufficiency and ascites. (a) CT shows typical density changes in the liver, suggesting Budd–Chiari syndrome. The hepatic veins were dilated, suggesting a weblike ostial stenosis. (b) Phlebography of the right hepatic vein confirms a tight, short stenosis located at the ostium. (c) A 10 mm Wallstent endoprosthesis was placed and PTA was performed inside the stent. Notice the persistent waist of the balloon (arrow) caused by the web. (d) Good flow was achieved in the hepatic vein after stenting. (e) Radiographs taken 2 years later show complete expansion of the stent. The patient is asymptomatic and Doppler confirmed stent patency.

(a)

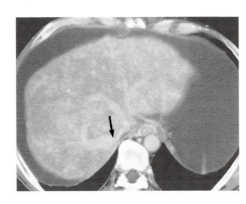

(b)

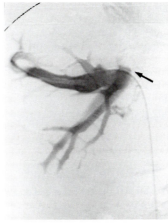

(c)

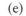

(d)

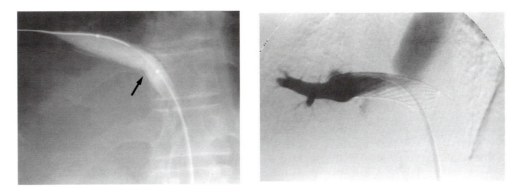

(e)

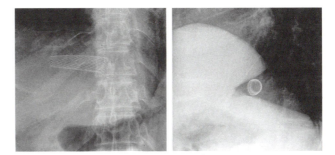

in the dominant, usually the right, hepatic vein only. In the 6 patients with a type II obstruction reported by Park *et al.*,[47] restenosis developed in 2, after a follow-up of 6 months to 6 years, and intimal thickening was found on cavography in all patients. Of the 33 cases reported by Wang *et al.*,[42] 24 were treated by stents alone. There was an excellent clinical result in all but one, 6–23 months following treatment. It is not clear if patients should be maintained on thrombolytic infusion for several days after stent placement, or on anticoagulants for a longer time period. Reduction of the caval diameter by 3–5 mm was observed after a 21-month follow-up, and did not progress to occlusive stenosis.[47] It has been suggested that intimal thickening is less pronounced and occurs later with an open stent configuration, such as the Gianturco stent.[38] Protrusion of stents placed in hepatic veins into the IVC may cause technical difficulties during liver transplantation.[48] The risk–benefit ratio must be taken into consideration for each patient. The main indication for stenting is restenosis or recoil following PTA; as angioplasty is frequently unsuccessful, stents should be inserted without delay when this procedure fails.

The hepatic veins are catheterized via a femoral or a jugular approach, depending on the angulation of the hepatic vein with the IVC. A percutaneous transhepatic approach or a rendezvous technique can be used in some cases of BCS to cross a tough web located at the ostium of a hepatic vein, when it cannot be entered by retrograde catheterization. The technique of transhepatic catheterization of the hepatic veins is similar to that used for percutaneous cholangiography, either blindly or with ultrasound guidance. A right transcapsular puncture is performed using a 22 gauge needle, and contrast medium is injected during needle withdrawal. When the hepatic vein is opacified, a 0.014 inch guidewire can be advanced through the hepatic vein stenosis into the IVC, and then snared and brought out through a sheath placed in the jugular vein. Stents can then be placed across the stenosis by the pull–push technique, which stabilizes the guidewire and catheter at both ends.

TIPS is another technique for treating BCS in selected patients with advanced disease, when no hepatic vein lumen is identifiable beyond the ostium.

Haemodialysis fistulae

Stenoses occurring in the peripheral or central venous outflow of haemodialysis fistulae, like most benign venous stenoses, respond poorly to PTA alone. Despite the use of local thrombectomy, high dose or pulse-spray thrombolysis and crossover infusion using two catheters, restenoses and rethromboses remain frequent, requiring repeat interventions at short time intervals. In cases of central venous stenoses related to haemodialysis fistulae, a 1-year patency rate of 0–35% has been demonstrated, the poorest results being seen with peripheral stenoses.[67,68] Primary placement of metal stents remains infrequent, as there are no significant data to support it. Stents are reserved for patients in whom PTA has failed because of recoil, or in whom stenosis has recurred. Probing of the stenosis with high-pressure balloons before stent placement is mandatory. Stents which are flexible, short, and with a minimal metal surface are probably the most suitable for these lesions. However, results are not particularly encouraging: a 40% 1-year patency has been reported in central stenoses, and a 2-year patency of 25% in both central and peripheral stenoses. As in TIPS, there is a need for frequent reinterventions (Fig. 2.8) to maintain patency.[33,36]

Figure 2.8

63-year-old female on haemodialysis. She experienced pain in the neck and left scapular region during each session of haemodialysis in March 1994. (a) Phlebography shows a concentric irregular, short segment stenosis in the left innominate vein (arrow) and reflux of contrast in the left jugular vein. (b) The stenosis did not respond to PTA and was therefore stented with two Wallstent endoprostheses (16 mm in diameter) (arrow) by a right femoral approach. (c) The stenosis (arrow) recurred inside the Wallstent endoprosthesis in May 1995. (d) Good flow was achieved after PTA with a 10 mm balloon. Notice the overlapping position of the Wallstent endoprostheses (arrow). (e) A regular narrowing (arrow), caused by tissue proliferation, recurred inside the stent in November 1995. (f) The stenosis (arrow) responded well to PTA. (g) The patient became symptomatic again in February 1996, and a recurrent stenosis (arrow) was seen in the same location. (h) The stenosis responded well again (arrow) to PTA.

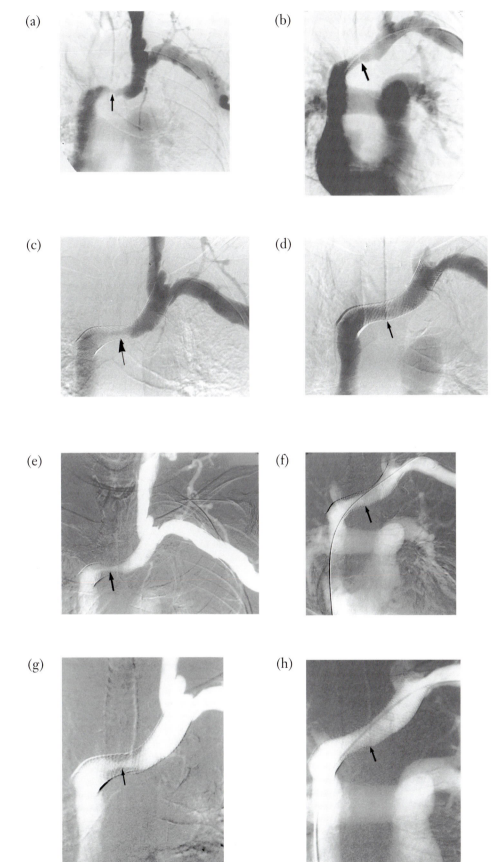

Personal experience

Twenty-six benign venous stenoses were treated in 24 patients. There were 12 males and 12 females with a mean age at treatment of 53.4 years (range: 29–73). No radiation-induced and no peripheral dialysis-related stenoses were included. Sixteen SVC stenoses were related to central venous catheters, and 2 subclavian stenoses were associated with mechanical compression. In 1 patient an SVC stenosis was caused by fibrosing mediastinitis. In 3 cases the cause was unclear. Two IVC stenoses were caused by BCS, 1 due to benign retroperitoneal fibrosis (Ormond disease), and 1 due to polycystic liver disease (Fig. 2.9). There was a technical failure in 1 patient with a very tight SVC stenosis secondary to post-traumatic fibrosing mediastinitis (Fig. 2.10). Immediate successful stent placement was achieved in 21 patients (88%). Initial stent placement was unsuccessful in 4 cases of subclavian vein stenosis, resulting in reobstruction. The thoracic outlet syndrome is not usually an indication for stent placement; however, stenting proved useful in 1 patient with extreme deformities due to ankylosing spondylitis and bilateral subclavian vein stenosis caused by clavicular compression. Symptomatic relief was obtained in all patients after proper stent placement. Primary stent patency was 72% after an average follow-up of 16 months (1–46). Reintervention consisting of PTA and placement of additional stents was required in 6 cases. These interventions were performed at an average of 8 months after primary stent placement. There was 1 case of obstruction after 18 months despite reintervention; thus secondary patency was 80%.

Complications

Complications related to venous stenting are relatively few. One death has been reported during placement of multiple stents in the IVC. Another death, from retroperitoneal bleeding, has been reported as a complication of anticoagulation.[23] Misplacement or stent migration are the most feared potential complications. Repositioning of a fully opened caval stent that has slipped beyond the stenosis is almost impossible. Stents should be long enough to cover the stenosis entirely. Stents with a too small diameter are prone to migration, even hours after placement.[64] Guidewires or catheters caught inside the mesh of the stent can cause displacement, even several weeks after stenting. Stents that have migrated to the heart or the pulmonary arteries should be removed using a snare or endovascular forceps to prevent trauma to the cardiac valves and endothelium (Fig. 2.11). A limited venotomy may be necessary for extraction of the stent at the femoral puncture site. Heparinization during the procedure avoids acute SVC thrombosis. Pulmonary oedema, attributable to volume overload caused by reperfusion, has been reported.[20] Stent thrombosis caused by external compression and paralysis of the median nerve following compression by a stent has also been observed.[33] Stent fragmentation has been observed with Gianturco stents; the authors have seen fragmentation and fraying of Wallstent endoprostheses placed in subclavian veins (Fig. 2.12). Caval perforation or mediastinal bleeding have not been reported. There are no reports of immediate surgery being necessary to deal with caval stent placement. Stent infection, bacteraemia, septicaemia and shock are potential complications; they should be minimized by the use of strict aseptic technique. Death secondary to sepsis in

Figure 2.9
73-year-old male with polycystic liver disease. The patient presented with sudden onset of oedema of both lower limbs. (a) Inferior cavography was performed by a right jugular approach. External compression of the retrohepatic IVC and massive clots in the caudal IVC are shown. (b) Catheterization of the right hepatic vein shows a pseudo Budd–Chiari syndrome caused by compression of the hepatic vein (arrow) by hepatic cysts. (c) Five double Z-stents (diameter: 2 cm; length: 5 cm) were placed in the IVC by a jugular approach, and dilated with a 10 mm balloon. The stents covered the ostia of the hepatic veins. Local thrombolysis was then started, using urokinase at an infusion rate of 75,000 IU/h, and continued for 3 days. (d) Cavography shows optimal caval flow following stenting and local thrombolysis. The patient became asymptomatic.

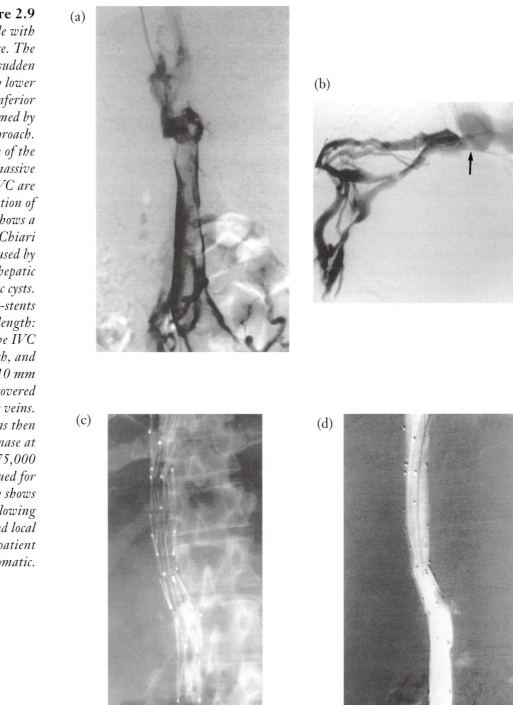

(a)

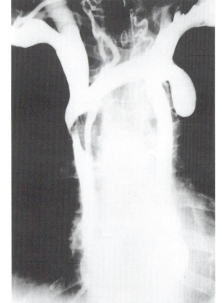

(b)

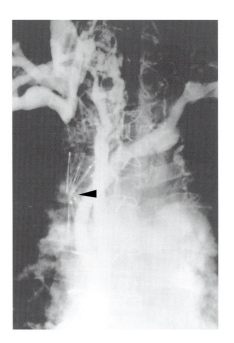

(c)

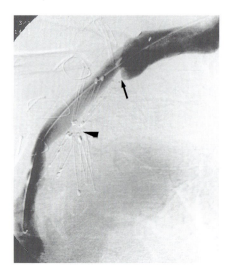

(d)

Figure 2.10

46-year-old healthy male presenting with a progressive superior vena cava syndrome. (a) Superior cavography confirmed a short tunnel-shaped stenosis of the SVC, caused by fibrosing mediastinitis, secondary to a mediastinal haematoma 15 years before. (b) A double Z-stent 2 cm in diameter was placed in the SVC stenosis (arrowhead), but did not expand. The SVC thrombosed and the patient underwent a surgical left innominate vein – right atrium bypass. (c) Five years later, the patient was again moderately symptomatic. Phlebography shows a moderate stenosis at the proximal anastomosis (arrow) and in the distal segment of the graft. (d) PTA was performed using a 10 mm balloon (arrow). The patient became symptom-free again. Notice the non-expanded Z-stent in the SVC.

Figure 2.11

60-year-old male with extreme deformity of the thorax caused by ankylosing spondylitis. The patient complained of swelling of both arms. (a) Phlebography of the left upper limb shows compression of the left subclavian vein, which is characteristic of a thoracic outlet syndrome (arrow). A Wallstent endoprosthesis (diameter: 10 mm; length: 3.5 cm) was placed by a left brachial approach. The stent migrated to the left pulmonary artery, several minutes after release (arrowheads). (b) Another Wallstent endoprosthesis (diameter: 10 mm; length: 7 cm) was placed in the subclavian vein. Improved flow was shown on phlebography. Notice the foreign body in the left pulmonary artery (arrowheads). (c) This Wallstent endoprosthesis was retrieved percutaneously using a goose-neck catheter (arrowhead), introduced by a right femoral approach.

(a)
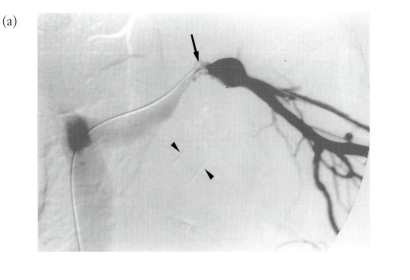

(b)
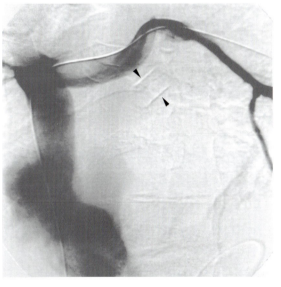

(c)
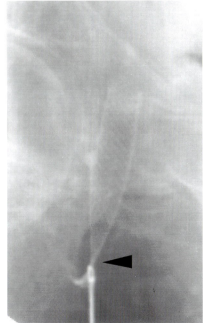

(a)

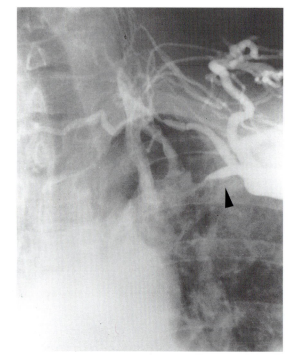

(b)

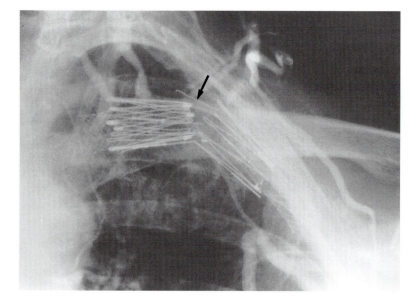

Figure 2.12
69-year-old female presenting with thrombosis of the left subclavian vein, probably caused by a venous line. (a) Phlebography of the left arm confirmed subclavian vein thrombosis (arrowhead). (b) The patient was treated with local urokinase infusion, and placement of a Gianturco stent (diameter: 1.5 cm; length: 5 cm) in a subclavian vein stenosis. The stent disintegrated (arrow), due to external compression by the clavicle, and thrombosis recurred. A 10 mm Wallstent endoprosthesis was then placed inside the Z-stent following repeated local thrombolysis. Phlebography performed 9 months later shows obstruction and fragmentation of both stents.

haemodialysis patients was reported before the use of prophylactic antibiotics.[26] The usual complications that may occur at the puncture site are seen: venous thrombosis, arteriovenous fistula and venous pseudoaneurysm. Nerve deficits have also been reported following peripheral stent placement in haemodialysis patients.[27]

References

1 Sherry CS, Diamond NG, Meyers TB, Martin RL. Successful treatment of superior vena cava syndrome by venous angioplasty. *Am J Roentgenol* 1986; **147**: 834–835.

2 Copek P, Cope C. Percutaneous treatment of superior vena cava syndrome. *Am J Roentgenol* 1989; **152**: 183–184.

3 Zeitler E. PTR in iliac vein thrombosis. In: Zeitler E, Grüntzig A, Schoop W (eds) *Percutaneous vascular recanalization*. Berlin, Springer Verlag, 1978; 145–147.

4 Yamada R, Sato M, Kawabata M *et al*. Segmental obstruction of the hepatic inferior vena cava treated by transluminal angioplasty. *Radiology* 1983; **49**: 91–96.

5 Jeans WK, Bourne JT, Read AE. Treatment of hepatic vein and inferior vena caval obstruction by balloon dilatation. *Br J Radiol* 1983; **56**: 687–689.

6 Uflaker R, Francisconi CF, Rodriguez MP *et al*. Percutaneous transluminal angioplasty of the hepatic veins for treatment of Budd–Chiari syndrome. *Radiology* 1984; **153**: 641–642.

7 Saced M, Newman GE, McCavin RL *et al*. Stenoses in dialysis fistulas: treatment with percutaneous angioplasty. *Radiology* 1987; **164**: 693–697.

8 Glanz S, Gordon DH, Lipkowitz GS *et al*. Axillary and subclavian vein stenosis: percutaneous angioplasty. *Radiology* 1980; **168**: 371–373.

9 Martin LG, Henderson JM, Millikan MJ *et al*. Angioplasty for long-term treatment of patients with Budd–Chiari syndrome. *Am J Roentgenol* 1990; **154**: 1007–1010.

10 Bernstein EF, Knowles HJ, Saced M. Should superior vena cava syndrome be treated by surgery any more? *Cardiovasc Surg* 1994; **2**: 605–606.

11 Maas D, Zollikofer CL, Largiader F, Senning A. Radiological follow-up of transluminally inserted vascular endoprostheses: an experimental study using expanding spirals. *Radiology* 1984; **152**: 659–663.

12 Charnsangavej C, Carrasco H, Wallace S *et al*. Stenosis of the vena cava: preliminary assessment of treatment with expandable metallic stents. *Radiology* 1986; **161**: 295–298.

13 Mullins CE, O'Laughlin MP, Vick GW *et al*. Implantation of balloon-expandable grafts by catheterization in pulmonary arteries and systemic veins. *Circulation* 1988; **77**: 188–189.

14 Parsson H, Norgren L, Ivancev K *et al*. Thrombogenicity of metallic vascular stents in arteries and veins: an experimental study in pigs. *Eur J Vasc Surg* 1990; **4**: 617–623.

15 Lopyan KS, Cross FL, Shoenfeld R *et al*. Use of the Medtronic-Wiktor stent in the venous system (abstract). *Radiology* 1990; **177** (P): 151.

16 Neville RF Jr, Bartorelli AL, Sidawy AN, Leon MB. Vascular stent deployment in vein bypass grafts: observations in an animal model. *Surgery* 1994; **116**: 55–61.

17 Rösch J, Bedell JE, Putnam J *et al*. Gianturco expandable wire stents in the treatment of superior vena cava syndrome recurring after maximum tolerance radiation. *Cancer* 1987; **60**: 1243–1246.

18 Putnam JS, Uchida BT, Antonovic R, Rösch J. Superior vena cava syndrome associated with massive thrombosis: treatment with expandable wire stents. *Radiology* 1988; **167**: 727–728.

19 Furui S, Sawada S, Kuramoto K *et al*. Gianturco stent placement in malignant caval obstruction: analysis of factors for predicting the outcome. *Radiology* 1995; **195**: 147–152.

20 Rösch J, Uchida BD, Hall LD *et al*. Gianturco–Rösch expandable Z stents in the treatment of superior vena cava syndrome. *Cardiovasc Intervent Radiol* 1992; **15**: 319–327.

21 Oudkerk M, Heystraten FM, Stoler G. Stenting in malignant vena caval obstruction. *Cancer* 1993; **71**: 142–146.

22 Irving JD, Dondelinger RF, Reidy JF *et al*. Gianturco self-expanding stents: clinical experience in the vena cava and large veins. *Cardiovasc Intervent Radiol* 1992; **15**: 328–333.

23 Dondelinger RF, Goffette P, Kurdziell JC, Roche A. Expandable metal stents for stenoses of the venae cavae and large veins. *Semin Intervent Radiol* 1991; **8**: 252–263.

24 Kishi K, Sonomura T, Mitsuzane K *et al*. Self-expandable metallic stent therapy for superior vena cava syndrome: clinical observations. *Radiology* 1993; **189**: 531–535.

25 Elson JD, Becker GJ, Wholey MH, Ehrman KO. Vena caval and central venous stenoses: management with Palmaz balloon-expandable intraluminal stents. *J Vasc Intervent Radiol* 1992; **2**: 215–223.

26 Tacke J, Antonucci F, Stuckmann G *et al*. The palliative treatment of venous stenoses in tumor patients with self-expanding vascular prostheses. *ROFO* 1994; **100**: 433–440.

27 Gaines PA, Belli AM, Anderson PB *et al*. Superior vena caval obstruction managed by the Gianturco Z stent. *Clin Radiol* 1994; **49**: 202–208.

28 Carlson JW, Nazarian GK, Hartenbach E *et al*. Management of pelvic venous stenosis with intravascular stainless steel stents. *Gynecol Oncol* 1995; **56**: 362–369.

29 Entwisle KG, Watkinson AF, Hibbert J, Adam A. The use of Wallstent endovascular prosthesis in the treatment of malignant inferior vena cava obstruction. *Clin Radiol* 1995; **50**: 310–313.

30 Furui S, Sawada S, Irie T *et al*. Hepatic inferior vena cava obstruction: treatment of two types with Gianturco expandable metallic stents. *Radiology* 1990; **176**: 620–621.

31 Antonucci F, Salomonowitz E, Stuckmann G *et al*. Hemodialysis related venous stenoses: treatment with self-expanding endovascular prostheses. *Eur J Radiol* 1992; **14**: 195–200.

32 Shoenfeld R, Hermans H, Novick A *et al*. Stenting of proximal venous obstructions to maintain hemodialysis access. *J Vasc Surg* 1994; **19**: 532–538.

33 Quinn SF, Schuman ES, Hall L *et al*. Venous stenoses in patients who undergo hemodialysis: treatment with self-expandable endovascular stents. *Radiology* 1992; **183**: 499–504.

34 Antonucci F, Salomonowitz E, Stuckmann G *et al*. Placement of venous stents: clinical experience with a self-expanding prosthesis. *Radiology* 1992; **183**: 493–497.

35 Ehrmann KO, Reed JD, Gaylord GM, Harris VM. Use of the Palmaz balloon-expandable stent in subclavian/brachiocephalic vein stenosis. *J Vasc Intervent Radiol* 1992; **3**: 13.

36 Vorwerk D, Aachen G, Guenther RW *et al*. Self-expanding stents in peripheral and central veins used for arteriovenous shunts: five years of experience. *Radiology* 1993; **189** (P): 174.

37 Zollikofer CL, Largiader I, Bruhlmaun WF *et al*. Endovascular stenting of veins and grafts: preliminary clinical experience. *Radiology* 1988; **167**: 707–712.

38 Nihill MR, Cooley DA. Successful stenting of a superior vena caval bypass graft. Report of a case. *Tex Heart Inst J* 1995; **22**: 105–106.

39 Bilba JI, Ruza M, Longo JM *et al*. Percutaneous transhepatic stenting by Wallstents of portal vein and bile duct stenoses caused by immunoblastic sarcoma in a liver transplantation. *Cardiovasc Intervent Radiol* 1994; **17**: 210–213.

40 Funaki B, Rosenblum JD, Leef JA *et al*. Portal vein stenosis in children with segmental liver transplants: treatment with percutaneous transhepatic venoplasty. *Am J Roentgenol* 1995; **165**: 161–165.

41 Dolmatch BL, Cooper BS, Chang PP *et al*. Percutaneous hepatic venous reanastomosis in a patient with Budd–Chiari syndrome. *Cardiovasc Intervent Radiol* 1995; **18**: 46–49.

42 Wang ZG, Wang SH, Wu JD. Treatment of Budd–Chiari syndrome with balloon dilatation and intraluminal stent. *Chung Hua I Hsueh Tsa Chih* 1995; **75**: 97–97.

43 Venbrux AC, Mitchell SE, Savander SJ *et al*. Long-term results with the use of metallic stents in the inferior vena cava for treatment of Budd–Chiari syndrome. *J Vasc Intervent Radiol* 1994; **5**: 411–416.

44 Lopez RR Jr, Benner KG, Hall L *et al*. Expandable venous stents for treatment of the Budd–Chiari syndrome. *Gastroenterology* 1991; **100**: 1435–1441.

45 Ishiguchi T, Fukatsu H, Itoh S *et al*. Budd–Chiari syndrome with long segmental inferior vena cava obstruction: treatment with thrombolysis, angioplasty and intravascular stents. *J Vasc Intervent Radiol* 1992; **3**: 421–425.

46 Walker HS, Rholl KS, Register TE, van Breda A. Percutaneous placement of a hepatic stent in the treatment of Budd–Chiari syndrome. *J Vasc Intervent Radiol* 1990; **1**: 23–27.

47 Park JH, Chung JW, Han JK, Han MC. Interventional management of benign obstruction of the hepatic inferior vena cava. *J Vasc Intervent Radiol* 1994; **5**: 403–409.

48 Martin L, Dondelinger RF, Trotteur G. Treatment of Budd–Chiari syndrome by metallic stent as a bridge to liver transplantation. *Cardiovasc Intervent Radiol* 1995; **18**: 196–199.

49 Fujimoto M, Moriyasu F, Someda H *et al*. Budd–Chiari syndrome recanalization of an occluded hepatic vein with percutaneous transluminal angioplasty and a metallic stent. *J Vasc Intervent Radiol* 1993; **4**: 257–261.

50 Gillams A, Dick R, Plattes A *et al*. Dilatation of the inferior vena cava using an expandable metal stent in Budd–Chiari syndrome. *J Hepatol* 1991; **13**: 149–151.

51 Berger A, Jaffe JW, York TN. Iliac compression syndrome treated with stent placement . *J Vasc Surg* 1995; **21**: 510–514.

52 Rosenblum J, Leef J, Messersmith R *et al*. Intravascular stents in the management of acute superior vena cava obstruction of benign etiology. *J Parenter Enteral Nutr* 1994; **18**: 362–366.

53 Abdulhamed JM, Al Youssef S, Khan MA, Mullins C. Balloon dilatation of complete obstruction of the superior vena cava after Mustard operation for transposition of great arteries. *Br Heart J* 1994; **72**: 482–485.

54 Dodds GA III, Harrison JK, O'Laughlin MP *et al*. Relief of superior vena cava syndrome, due to fibrosing mediastinitis using the Palmaz stent. *Chest* 1994; **1406**: 315–318.

55 Schlessinger AE, Caoili EM, Mendelson AM *et al*. Radiography of thoracic intravascular stents in children with congenital heart disease. *Pediatr Radiol* 1993; **23**: 113-116.

56 Marks MP, Dake MD, Steinberg GK *et al*. Stent placement for arterial and venous cerebrovascular disease: preliminary experience. *Radiology* 1994; **191**: 309–312.

57 Harrison DA, Berison LN, Cusimano RJ, MacLaughlin PR. Right-to-left shunt following repair of partial anomalous pulmonary venous connection: a novel use of the Rashkind double-umbrella occlusion device. *Cathet Cardiovasc Diagn* 1994; **33**: 361.

58 Francis CM, Starkey IR, Errington ML, Gillespie IN. Venous stenting as treatment for pacemaker-induced superior vena cava syndrome. *Am Heart J* 1995; **29**: 836–837.

59 Schraufnagel DE, Hill R, Leech JA, Parc JAP. Superior vena caval obstruction: is it a medical emergency ? *Am J Med* 1981; **70**: 1169–1174.

60 Schoch EG, Pfyffer M, Figi T, Zollikofer CL. Microporous angioplasty balloon: new method for local thrombolysis of acute and subacute arterial occlusion. *Radiology* 1994; **193** (P) : 163.

61 Grimm W, Schwieder R, Wagner T. Deep vein thrombosis: methods of thrombolytic therapy compared. *Biomed Prog* 1994; **7**: 3–7.

62 Kamalesh M, Stokes K, Burger AJ. Transesophageal echocardiography assisted retrieval of embolized inferior vena cava stent. *Cathet Cardiovasc Diagn* 1994; **33**: 178–180.

63 Ge S, Shiota T, Rice MJ *et al*. Images in cardiovascular medicine. Transesophageal ultrasound imaging during stent implantation to relieve superior vena cava-to-intra-atrial baffle obstruction after mustard repair of transposition of the great arteries. *Circulation* 1995; **91**: 2679–2680.

64 Bartorelli AL, Fabbiocchi F, Montorsi P *et al*. Successful transcatheter management of Palmaz stent embolization after superior vena caval stenting. *Cathet Cardiovasc Diagn* 1995; **34**: 162–166.

65 Trerotola SO. Interventional Radiology in central venous stenosis and occlusion. *Semin Intervent Radiol* 1994; **11**: 291–304.

66 Martin L, Dondelinger RF. The treatment of Budd–Chiari syndrome by percutaneous transluminal angioplasty. *Rev Im Med* 1993; **6**: 31–36.

67 Glanz S, Gordon DH, Butt KMH *et al*. The role of percutaneous angioplasty in the management of chronic hemodialysis fistulas. *Ann Surg* 1987; **206**: 777–781.

68 Beathard GA. Percutaneous transvenous angioplasty in the treatment of vascular access stenosis. *Kidney Int* 1992; **42**: 1390–1397.

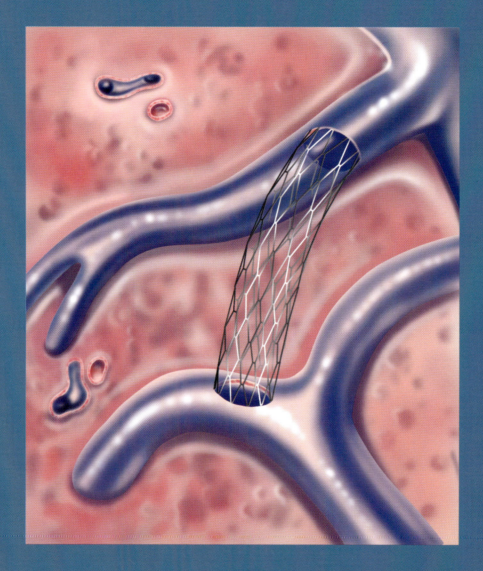

Chapter 3

Transjugular intrahepatic portosystemic shunt (TIPS)

H. Rousseau, J.P. Vinel, J. El-Khoury, P. Otal, K. Barange, P. Maquin and F. Joffre

Introduction

Approximately one-third of all deaths of patients with cirrhosis of the liver is caused by bleeding from ruptured oesophagogastric varices, secondary to portal hypertension (PHT).[1] In the past, surgical decompression was considered the most effective treatment of the complications of PHT. However, because of the high operative mortality rate (particularly following emergency surgery), the potential occurrence of chronic encephalopathy, and the fact that surgery has not been shown to increase long-term survival, it has decreased in popularity over the last few years. Currently, endoscopic sclerosis (or ligation) is the most widely used therapy for the achievement of haemostasis and the prevention of rebleeding. Haemostasis is achieved in more than 90% of patients. The remaining 10% fail to respond and are candidates for complementary therapy.[2–5] Haemorrhage may result in patients in whom the varices have not been completely eradicated.

The limitations of surgery and sclerotherapy motivated the search for a safer and more efficient means for lowering portal pressure. The ideal therapy should lower portal pressure enough to control bleeding and ascites without causing encephalopathy. This can be achieved by creating a hepatic portosystemic anastomosis. Initially, transjugular intrahepatic portosystemic shunt (TIPS) was considered a panacea for all types of patients and the technique was used indiscriminately; in the light of subsequent experience, TIPS is now more appropriately used in specific, selected cases with portal hypertension.

Historical review

A radiologically created intrahepatic fistula between a hepatic vein and a major branch of the portal vein was first envisioned by Rösch and Hanafee in 1968 when, while performing experimental transjugular cholangiography, they opacified the portal venous system. In 1969, Rösch et al. published the first experimental results describing a radiologically created anastomosis between the right hepatic vein and right branch of the portal vein.[6,7] A new concept was born, but at this time the technical components necessary to perform the procedures (guidewires, catheters, stents) were not available. Ten years later, with the development of metallic endovascular endoprostheses, further experimentation and creation of these shunts became possible.[8] Palmaz in 1985, and Rösch in

1987, demonstrated in animal studies that it was possible to create and maintain a portacaval anastomosis by using the Palmaz™ (Johnson & Johnson, Warren, NJ, USA) and Gianturco™ (William Cook Europe, Denmark) metallic endoprostheses.[9,10] However, they noted that, in healthy animals without PHT, the anastomosis was transient and the intrahepatic tract was progressively occluded by hepatic tissue proliferation and local thrombosis. Palmaz noted[11] that, in animals in which PHT was induced experimentally, there was increased patency of the radiologically placed shunts, perhaps due to increased flow through the prosthesis. Both authors demonstrated that the metallic prosthesis would eventually be covered by a non-thrombogenic surface composed of a 1–1.5 mm thick neointima of endothelium. Similar experimental results were also observed with the Wallstent™ (Schneider, AG, Bulach, Switzerland) prosthesis (Fig. 3.1).[12] These encouraging experimental data prompted the first clinical application of TIPS by Richter in 1988.[13] Soon after, the TIPS procedure, as it was called, gained worldwide popularity and numerous clinical trials were started.

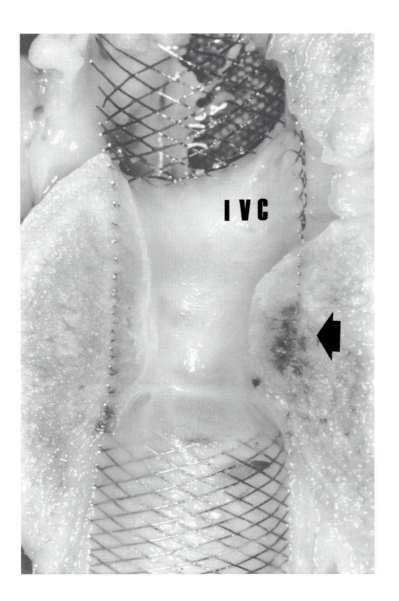

Figure 3.1
Histological results obtained with a Wallstent prosthesis implanted in a pig. When an experimental PHT is created, the prosthesis is covered by a neointima (arrowhead) with an endothelial layer, preventing subsequent thrombosis (arrowhead = small area of hepatic tissue proliferation through metallic filament) (IVC: inferior vena cava).

Technical aspects

Preoperative preparation

Occasionally, in some centres, general anaesthesia is used. TIPS is a relatively safe procedure and in most cases can be performed with intravenous analgesia. Except in emergency cases, coagulation factors can usually be corrected to reduce the risk of intraperitoneal haemorrhage, which is the major complication of this procedure. The authors give prophylactic antibiotics with a limited effect on hepatic metabolism, usually fluoroquinolones (200 mg) intravenously. They often use colour-Doppler ultrasonography before the shunt to verify patency of the portal vein and to analyse hepatic and vascular morphology. Ultrasound can also be used to determine the ideal route for vascular access and to evaluate the size and calibre of the hepatic and portal veins, as well as the intrahepatic tract length. Some authors advocate the use of spiral CT for this morphological evaluation.

Procedure

The technique for performance of a TIPS procedure is well described.[14–17] The right internal jugular vein is almost always used, although on occasion the external jugular, left internal jugular or the femoral vein could be cannulated for the procedure.[18] However, these latter veins are usually very tortuous, which results in technical difficulties; they should be chosen only when the right internal jugular vein is thrombosed or not possible to use.

After insertion of the guidewire, the authors prefer to use a long introducer (35 cm, 10 Fr) (Cook). Placement of the introducer into the hepatic vein straightens the tract and makes the transhepatic puncture of the portal vein easier. The introducer is placed into a hepatic vein of sufficient calibre and low angulation with the inferior cava. In most instances they choose the right main hepatic vein. In rare cases, when the hepatic veins are absent or when it proves impossible to align the hepatic and portal veins, a transcaval anastomosis can be performed by direct puncture of the inferior vena cava in its retrohepatic portion (Fig. 3.2).

Localizing the portal vein

Various techniques have been described for puncture of the portal vein:

1 Richter *et al.* first described a direct puncture of the portal vein through a transhepatic approach.[13] This is not currently recommended because of the high risk of intraperitoneal haemorrhage. Others have suggested using ultrasound guidance to localize the portal vein and guide percutaneous placement of 'platinum' guidewires at the portal bifurcation. This is a relatively straightforward technique in the absence of ascites and in patients with normal liver size.

2 Localization of the portal vein by direct mesenteric angiography has disadvantages and is not commonly used: angiography requires a second invasive procedure and can lead to iodine overload; however, it has been advocated in patients with severe hepatic atrophy.

3 Ultrasound can also be used to guide needles percutaneously into the portal vein by direct puncture.[19] This method has been useful in patients who have hepatic atrophy, ascites and portal vein thrombosis. The major disadvantage of

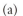

(a)

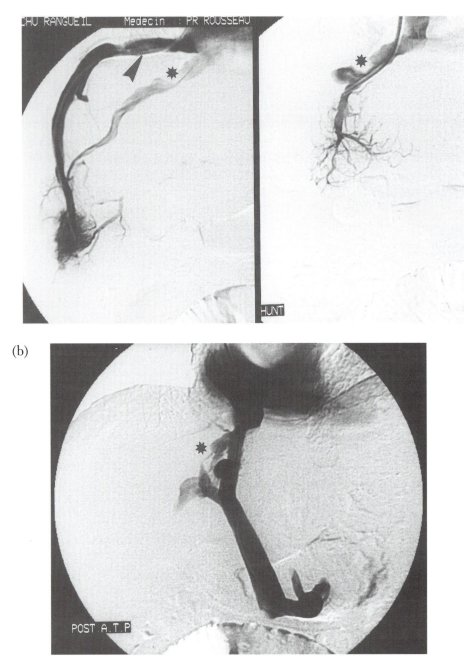

(b)

Figure 3.2
For TIPS placement, a hepatic vein of sufficient calibre and low angulation with inferior vena cava must be chosen. (a) The right main hepatic vein is suitable in most cases, but in this case angulation of the main hepatic vein makes shunt creation impossible (arrowhead). (b) TIPS creation was performed with another hepatic vein, close to the vena cava to avoid a proximal hepatic vein stenosis (star).

this technique is that the hands of the operator may be directly in the X-ray beam.

The authors' preferred method of guidance is to advance an Amplatz (Cook) guidewire into the hepatic vein, to visualize its position with fluoroscopy, and then guide the transhepatic needle into the portal vein.

4   Another simple way to visualize the portal vein is with wedged hepatic venography. Using this method, the authors can opacify the portal vein adequately in approximately 70% of cases. After the catheter has been wedged into a major hepatic vein, 20 ml contrast material is injected at a rate of 6 ml/s (Fig. 3.3). Other authors have suggested the use of CO_2 to facilitate the transsinusoidal crossing.

Figure 3.3
Wedged hepatic venography is performed by injecting 20 ml contrast material at a rate of 6 ml/s, the catheter being deeply blocked in a major hepatic vein. This simple method demonstrates portal vein anatomy, which is very useful in guiding portal puncture (arrows indicate direction of flow).

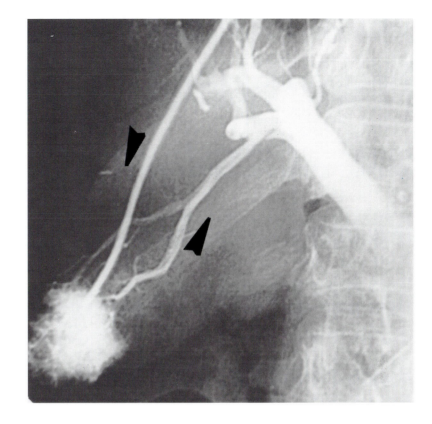

5 Catheterization and opacification of the umbilical vein has also been suggested.

6 Finally, many individuals perform a blind portal puncture under fluoroscopic control. General anatomical landmarks can be used to help facilitate this procedure. In most patients, in a standard anteroposterior position the portal bifurcation is located between the 11th and 12th ribs, approximately 4 cm away from the lateral vertebral edge.[20]

The authors have found wedged hepatic venography to be a useful method of guiding portal puncture. Ultrasonography is used as the guidance method in cases in which technical difficulties are encountered.

Puncture technique

Once the portal system has been located, the needle is placed in the hepatic vein over an Amplatz guidewire. The needle is then slowly withdrawn until it is 2–3 cm away from the junction with the inferior vena cava. A rapid counterclockwise rotation of approximately 90° is then applied to the needle, which is directed towards the anatomical landmarks described above. The transhepatic needle penetrates approximately 2–4 cm into hepatic parenchyma to reach the portal vein. Ideally, the right vein should be punctured. Puncture of the portal bifurcation or the main portal vein can result in intraperitoneal bleeding. The needle is then slowly withdrawn and its position is verified by injecting contrast material. A guidewire is then advanced via the needle into the splenic or superior mesenteric vein. Following this, a catheter can be advanced coaxially over the needle guide.

A variety of different types of needles can be used for the TIPS procedure:

1   A regular or Colapinto needle (16 G);[21]
2   A Rösch needle composed of a 5 Fr catheter with a coaxial guidewire which
    can be placed through a 14 G needle. The main advantage of this needle is
    that it allows performance of the transhepatic puncture with a relatively small-
    calibre catheter. Its main disadvantage lies in the fact that it is quite flexible,
    making puncture difficult in fibrotic livers.
3   The Richter needle (Angiomed-Bard, Karlsruhe, Germany) has also been
    described. Its tip is echogenic, and its relative stiffness makes puncture easier.
    On the other hand, the stiffness of the needle makes manoeuvrability difficult,
    resulting in rather central punctures, near the portal bifurcation.

Once the portal system has been catheterized, the portacaval pressure gradient
can be measured. Prior to deployment of the endoprosthesis, a 10 mm balloon
dilatation catheter is placed through the intrahepatic tract, bridging the portal
vein and hepatic venous systems. Inflation of the balloon usually demonstrates a
waist at the entrance of the portal and hepatic veins. After dilatation has been
accomplished and the waist has been abolished, the endoprosthesis can be placed.
The ideal position is to have the endoprosthesis bridge the whole tract between
the portal branch and hepatic veins.

Once the prosthesis is released, a direct contrast portogram can be performed
to evaluate the calibre and patency of the shunt and to check the flow direction of
the blood. The portacaval pressure gradient is measured again to evaluate the
efficiency of the shunt. Repeat dilatation of the prosthesis is performed with a
larger balloon, if the portacaval pressure gradient is above 12 mmHg and/or if
there is persistent opacification of collateral vessels on portography. If collateral
vessels continue to fill, direct embolization can be performed.

Stent type

The two most common types of protheses used are the Palmaz and the Wallstent
endoprosthesis. The Palmaz prosthesis is balloon expandable, and its diameter can
be changed with larger balloons. This is particularly helpful in patients who have a
high residual portal pressure after initial placement. The disadvantage of the Palmaz
prosthesis is its short length (3 cm) and its relative inflexibility. The Wallstent
prosthesis is a self-expanding stent that is available in different lengths. However, it
has a fixed diameter. The advantage of this stent is its flexibility, which is helpful in
traversing vascular curves. Its main disadvantages are its low radio-opacity and, more
important, its considerable shortening (35%) after placement. Other prostheses have
been described but these are still under evaluation. The Gianturco prosthesis is easy
to place, but can become kinked when implanted too laterally within the hepatic
parenchyma. The Strecker™ (Boston Scientific, Watertown, MA, USA) tantalum
balloon expandable prosthesis is both very flexible and radio-opaque, but has an
extremely small radial force, thus allowing a risk of peri-procedural migration.[22] The
Cragg (MinTec, Freeport, Grand Bahama) and Memotherm™ (Angiomed-Bard,
Karlsruhe, Germany) nitinol prostheses have some of the same advantages as the
Wallstent in that they are available in different lengths, are flexible and self-
expandable; however, they shorten to a much lesser degree than the Wallstent,
making their implantation more precise (Fig. 3.4 and Fig. 3.5).

Figure 3.4
Transjugular portosystemic anastomosis. Initial angiography showed clear portal flow derivation to left gastric veins. These derivation channels were no longer opacified after a Memotherm prosthesis was placed between a right portal vein branch and right hepatic vein. Advantages of the nitinol prostheses are many available lengths and diameters, good flexibility with, in addition, little shortening when released in place, making its implantation very precise.

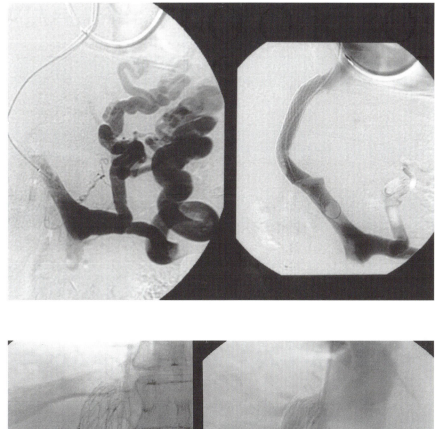

Figure 3.5
After a rebleeding episode, 10 days after a first right hepatic to right portal vein 10 mm TIPS, the pressure measurement demonstrated a portosystemic gradient at 17 mmHg, demonstrating that the first shunt was not large enough to decompress the portal venous system. Portogram obtained after placement of second right hepatic to left portal vein parallel TIPS (10 mm Cragg stent) demonstrates excellent flow through both shunts and no evidence of variceal filling. The final portosystemic gradient was 11 mmHg

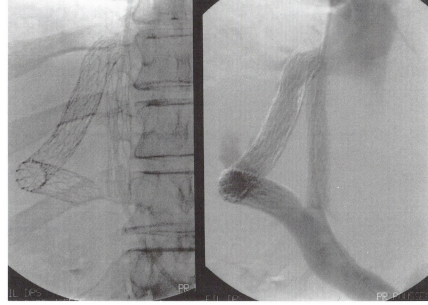

Follow-up

Clinical and radiological follow-up after placement of a portacaval prosthesis is mandatory. However, there is no consensus on the optimal time schedule and method of follow-up. Many radiologists believe that colour-Doppler ultrasonography is the procedure of choice. It is non-invasive and enables excellent evaluation of: (1) the peak velocity and flow within the shunt; (2) the peak velocity in the portal vein; (3) the flow direction in the hepatic portal branches and hepatic vein; and (4) early detection of stent stenosis.[23–5] In most cases, the mean flow velocity measured initially after the procedure averages 123 cm/s. A 30% decrease of flow velocity is observed during the first

3 months; subsequently, it usually stabilizes. In approximately 2–40% of cases, the flow progressively decreases and actually reverses because of excessive intimal hyperplasia or hepatic vein stenosis. The most sensitive and significant sign of shunt failure is a fall in shunt flow peak velocity to values below 50 cm/s.[24] To date, Doppler ultrasonography is considered the gold standard examination for TIPS follow-up.[26] In equivocal cases, shunt opacification and pressure gradient measurements should be performed, before complete shunt thrombosis occurs.

Results (Tables 3.1 and 3.2)

Several retrospective studies comparing the Wallstent with the Palmaz prosthesis have suggested that the former is a better stent to use for the TIPS procedure because fewer stents are required to bridge the hepatic portal tract and fewer shunt-related complications have been observed following its use. However, a recent randomized, controlled study in 60 patients showed comparable early complications, occlusion, rebleeding and survival rates between the two stents.[27] Importantly, a recent multicentre study of 1750 TIPS reported in 1995 indicated a technical success of approximately 97%.[28] With experience, failure is rare. The causes of failure are usually anatomical (portal vein thrombosis, hepatic vein occlusion, major hepatic atrophy or massive ascites). Overall, the mean pressure gradient drop has been reported to be approximately 50% with a residual gradient of 10 mmHg.

Table 3.1
Subjects.

References	Rossle et al. (29)	Laberge et al. (14)	Helton et al. (30)	Jalan et al. (32)	Perarnau et al. (31)	Rousseau et al. (17)	Coldwell et al. (33)
No. of patients	100	100	59	64*	49	45	96
Age (years)	57	50	51	56	58	57	56
Type of stent used	Palmaz	Wallstent	Wallstent	34 Wallstent 24 Palmaz	Palmaz	Wallstent	Wallstent
Indications:							
Active bleeding	10	32	23	1	1	NA	48
Recurrent bleeding	90	62	34	44	44	36	48
Refractory ascites	–	3	2	3	3	9	
Others	–	3	–	1	1		
Child–Pugh (n)							
A	24	10	4	12	12	6	24
B	46	35	22	27	27	11	28
C	20	55	33	10	10	28	34
Follow-up (months)	12	4.7	NA	8	8	7.2	6

NA: not available
*The TIPS procedure was successful in 56 of the 64 patients in this study.

Table 3.2
Results.

References	Rossle *et al.* (29)	Laberge *et al.* (14)	Helton *et al.* (30)	Jalan *et al.* (32)	Perarnau *et al.* (31)	Rousseau *et al.* (17)	Coldwell *et al.* (33)
Procedure-related mortality rate (%)	1	0	5	3.1	2	2	2
Success rate (%)	93	96	93	87.5	94	94	100
Control bleeding	100	98	90	88.8	NA	100	100
Pressure gradient (mmHg)							
before TIPS	21	34.5	18.1	20.1	21	19.1	22.8
after TIPS	9.2	24.5	10.5	10.2	10	10	12.8
Variceal rebleeding (%)	22	19	39	22.7	12	22	16
TIPS obstruction (%)	33	16	18	28	39	31	27
Encephalopathy (%)	25	18	17	10.7	17	20	29
Survival at 6 months (%)	90	NA	NA	NA	88	67	NA

NA: not available

Results for variceal bleeding

In most published series, the TIPS procedure was successful in controlling haemorrhage from oesophageal varices in over 90% of patients.[14,17,29,30,31–3] However, many of these studies do not take into consideration other therapeutic means of controlling variceal bleeding, making the exact role of TIPS in these patients somewhat difficult to evaluate. More recent studies have shown that the efficacy approached 100% in patients with variceal bleeding treated on an emergency basis; however, there was a 60% mortality within the first month.[33,34] Overall, as reported in the multicentre study of 1750 TIPS procedures, the cumulative rebleeding rate was 5.6% (1 to 13%) at 9 months, 16.6% (2 to 26%) at 12 months, and 20.7% (5 to 29%) in long-term follow-up.[28] The rebleeding rates were twice as high in urgently treated patients.[30] In 10–22% of these cases, the haemorrhage originated from oesophageal varices occurring after shunt occlusion.[29]

The preliminary results of the first randomized prospective study comparing TIPS with sclerotherapy[35] showed similar recurrence rates (21 and 25%, respectively). However, there was a markedly higher mortality rate following TIPS (28 versus 11%; p < 0.005). These results are difficult to interpret owing to the small number of patients included in the study and the delay (up to 3 weeks) between the index bleed and inclusion in the study. More recent reports have suggested that the rebleeding rate was significantly lower in patients with TIPS as opposed to sclerotherapy, but no benefit in survival was noted (Table 3.3).[36–9] Comparison with sclerotherapy may be difficult because now variceal band ligation and clipping is becoming more popular.

Results for refractory ascites

Results for treatment of refractory ascites vary from one series to another.[40–3] However, the overall success rates are between 50 and 80% in most hands. The

References	TIPS			Sclerotherapy		
	No of patients	Rebleeding rate (%)	Death rate (%)	No of patients	Rebleeding rate (%)	Death rate (%)
Sanyal et al. (35)	40	23	28	39	15†	10†
Rossle et al. (36)	29	21	17	29	55†	17
Cabrera et al. (37)	23	13	13	23	30	9
Vinel et al.* (38)	34	41	47*	34	65	47*
Bezzi et al. (39)	29	13	13	29	25†	6
Total	155	22	23.6	154	38	17.8

* only in Child C
†p<0.05 (sclerotherapy vs TIPS)

Table 3.3
Results of five recent studies comparing rebleeding and death rates for TIPS and sclerotherapy.

differences may be due to the variety of numbers of patients included in each study as well as the varying definitions of refractory ascites.[44] A recently reported prospective study comparing TIPS with paracentesis in 25 patients demonstrated that after 4 months there was 100% success in ameliorating ascites in Child B type patients with TIPS, as compared with only 33% in patients who underwent paracentesis. There was, however, no difference recorded in Child C type patients. Interestingly, the 1-year survival was significantly lower in TIPS patients (17 versus 58%).[45] The major complication rate in patients treated for ascites has been reported to be approximately 32% and this is considerably higher than in patients who are treated primarily for haemorrhagic varices.[41] This could be explained by the technical difficulties due to the relatively small liver seen in these patients, and the worse haemodynamic status of patients with refractory ascites. Consequently, most authors feel that the use of TIPS for ascites should be restricted, and reserved for selected patients who are resistant to conventional treatment.

Complications

Early complications

The mortality during the first month after the TIPS procedure has been reported to vary between 2 and 13%.[14,17,29,35,46] This difference is most likely due to the different inclusion criteria in clinical staging of the patients in individual studies.[47] The early complication rate averages approximately 10% and is related to operator experience. Intraperitoneal haemorrhage is seen in 1–6% of cases, due to hepatic capsular puncture.[28] Other inadvertent catheter punctures have been reported, including puncture of the biliary tree, gallbladder and hepatic arterial branches, with no significant clinical consequences in most cases.[48,49] Most centres use pre-procedure systemic prophylactic antibiotics, despite the fact that infectious complications are rarely encountered. Less frequently reported complications include haemobilia, renal insufficiency, disseminated intravascular coagulation and intravascular haemolysis.[50]

Hepatic deterioration after a TIPS procedure is variable in most published series, but approximately one-third of patients have a transient worsening of liver function; a rapid deterioration of hepatic function should suggest a more serious problem such as an associated arterial lesion.[51] Because decompression of the portal system can result in a significant increase in right atrial pressure, acute pulmonary oedema with cardiac decompression has been reported. Prospective haemodynamic studies performed during TIPS have shown a rise in free and wedged pulmonary arterial pressure as well as a rise in cardiac output immediately after the procedure. Subsequently, pulmonary pressure returns to normal while cardiac output remains high in these patients; this results in a worsening of the hyperkinetic circulation that characterizes portal hypertension.[52] These findings seem to justify measurement of pulmonary pressure in high-risk patients, in order to treat potentially significant haemodynamic complications.

Secondary complications

The two most commonly encountered secondary complications are encephalopathy and delayed occlusion of the stent.

Encephalopathy occurs in 10–20% of cases and appears to be directly proportional to the age of the patient and the shunt diameter, and inversely proportional to serum albumin levels.[53,54] In most cases, encephalopathy is secondary to another complication such as recurrent haemorrhage, shunt stenosis or hepatic artery occlusion. Encephalopathy due to large shunt diameter usually regresses and declines with time because of the progressive reduction of shunt calibre by the physiological intimal proliferation over the prosthesis. Persistent encephalopathy, however, can be treated by embolization of the shunt or other methods to reduce the lumen. In many cases, encephalopathy can be controlled by medical treatment.

A randomized prospective study comparing TIPS with sclerotherapy reported that encephalopathy was significantly more frequent during the first week in patients treated with TIPS, while similar encephalopathy rates were recorded after a 3-month follow-up period.[55]

Shunt insufficiency

Shunt stenosis can be defined as a reduction of the diameter of the shunt of more than 50%, with a portacaval pressure gradient exceeding 15 mmHg. The incidence of secondary occlusion varies in different reports, but averages 30–40% after 12 months and 68% after 24-month follow-up.[17,29,48,56–8] This complication can be due to two different mechanisms: thrombosis and/or intimal hyperplasia. Occlusions in the first month can almost always be attributed to thrombosis and occur in 9–13% of cases. Most of these are due to technical problems such as prosthesis shortening, insufficient shunt calibre or a major angulation causing shunt stenosis. The use of anticoagulants and/or antiplatelet drugs does not seem to affect the occurrence of this complication.[59] However, many authors agree that Child A patients with normal coagulation factors could benefit from anticoagulants. After the first month, occlusions are usually secondary to excessive intimal hyperplasia, the mechanism of which is not completely clear.[56] Occlusion seems to be more frequent when the hepatic function is normal and when a major angulation is noted in the position of the shunt tract. No definite predictive factor has been identified, but biliary fistulae have been found both radiologically and histologically to be more frequent in patients with occluded shunts.[60]

The authors' group has performed a histopathological study correlating the angiographical and histological findings in 22 patients who had TIPS and were examined at either autopsy or transplantation. During the first week (4–8 days) there was evidence of moderate protrusion of hepatic parenchyma into the shunt lumen between the metal stent filaments.[61] The hepatic parenchyma remained compressed with no evidence of vascular thrombosis or biliary stasis, and few parenchymal haemorrhagic or necrotic areas were noted. Fibrin deposits of approximately 100 μm thickness were seen over the metallic filaments. At approximately one month, a new intima had formed, made up of collagen and granulomatous tissue and filled with capillary proliferation. This new intima covered the whole intraparenchymal tract, but seemed to be more developed in the middle section. After the first month, there was no evidence of hepatic parenchyma proliferation; the new intima contained more collagen fibres and fewer cellular elements, and was covered by endothelial cells (Fig. 3.6). This new intimal layer was found to be approximately 660 μm thick at 9 months.

It seems, then, that the prosthesis is covered early in its course with connective tissue overlaid with endothelium; this new intimal reaction demonstrates little development, except in a few cases where it continues to proliferate, eventually

(a)

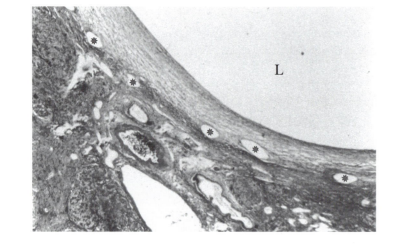

(b)

Figure 3.6
Histopathological study performed 6 months after TIPS implantation. (a) Optic microscopy study shows a regular intrahepatic lumen (L) covered with a neointima with high collagen content (stars = location of metallic filaments, removed to enable histopathological study). (b) Electromicroscopic study showing complete covering of this fibrous tissue by an endothelium.

occluding the shunt. Occlusions can occur anywhere along the shunt, but seem to predominate in the region of the hepatic veins. The exact mechanism of this excessive hyperplasia and hepatic vein stenosis remains obscure.

Whatever the cause, these occlusions can be treated percutaneously. Fibrinolysis, which has been advocated in acute thrombosis, does not seem to have a place in these patients who are at a high risk of bleeding. The most commonly performed procedure is angioplasty of the stenosed stent followed by implantation of a new prosthesis. In a patient who has significant stenosis, the Colapinto needle can be useful for catheterization of a completely occluded shunt. Creation of a second shunt should be considered whenever recanalization is not possible.

The restenosis rate increases with time; shunt patency averages 75, 50 and 32% at 6, 12 and 24 months, respectively. However, there are good long-term results after a second intervention. Haskal *et al.* described an 85% secondary patency rate at 1 year, versus 50% after a single intervention.[58] Likewise, Coldwell *et al.*, in a multicentre trial, reported a 33% reintervention rate in 100 TIPS patients; this averaged out at 0.5 reinterventions per patient. There was a 98% patency rate at 6 months, achieved with 1, 2, 3 or 4 reinterventions in 22, 8, 2 and 1% of cases, respectively.[33]

Indications

At present, most authors would agree that there are two major indications for performing the TIPS procedure:

Bleeding
In general, TIPS should not be used as the first line of therapy for patients with portal hypertension and haemorrhage. However, if the bleeding is refractory to the usual medical and/or endoscopic therapies, a TIPS procedure should be considered. Most authors feel that TIPS is preferable to surgery in patients with poor liver function and/or those candidates awaiting liver transplantation.

Refractory ascites
Patients resistant to diuretic treatment can benefit from the TIPS procedure. However, unlike refractory haemorrhage, where there are very few therapeutic options, recurrent ascites is not usually life threatening, and other methods of treatment, such as therapeutic paracentesis combined with volumetric compensation, can always be attempted. As there is a higher complication rate in this group of patients, a thorough pre-procedure evaluation is necessary, particularly in those patients with cardiac or renal insufficiency.

Liver transplantation

The authors feel strongly that the main indication for TIPS is the temporary relief of portal hypertension in patients awaiting liver transplantation.[62] Because the stent is placed intrahepatically, the shunt will be removed during the liver transplantation procedure and consequently should not affect the outcome of the transplant.

Other potential indications have been suggested: (1) gastric haemorrhage or haemorrhage caused by ectopic varices;[63] (2) portal hypertension associated with oesophageal or rectal tumours;[64] (3) treatment of thrombosed surgical portacaval

(a)

(b)

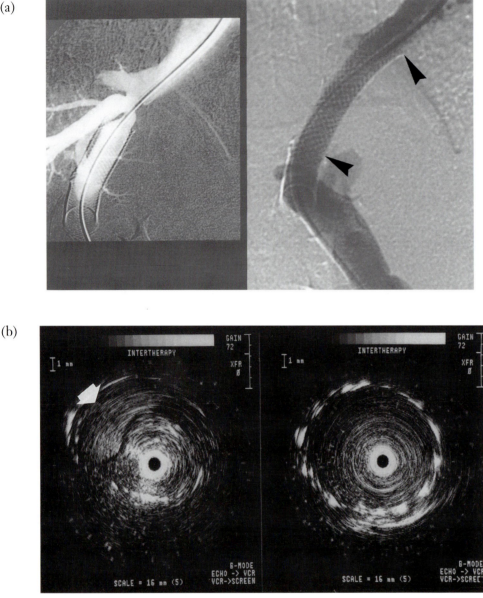

Figure 3.7
Restenosis in a 6-month-old prosthesis implanted between right branch of portal vein and right hepatic vein. (a) Portocaval pressure gradient measured 25 mmHg before and 13 mmHg after the stenosis was dilated and a second prosthesis (arrowheads) was implanted to restore a satisfactory hepatic tract diameter. (b) Endovascular ultrasonography demonstrates an intimal proliferation (arrowhead) inside the proximal part of the stent and a good patency of the shunt after stent insertion. Intraportal ultrasound (US) can provide more valuable information than using only direct portography or colour-Doppler US, in determining the exact position of the prosthesis inside the portal and the hepatic vein, the size of the path inside the parenchyma and the thickness of the intimal hyperplasia inside the stent during the follow-up.

anastomosis or encephalopathy after surgical shunts;[17] (4) Budd–Chiari syndrome;[65–7] and (5) hydrothorax (Fig. 3.8).[68]

Contraindications

Polycystic liver disease and hepatocellular carcinoma are the main contraindications. Relative contraindications include encephalopathy, portal thrombosis, infection, and cardiorespiratory, renal or hepatic failure. Portal thrombosis is not an absolute contraindication; however, it may complicate the TIPS procedure. An acute or chronic portal thrombosis can be recanalized and treated by a prosthesis placed in the portal vein. If the thrombosis is recent, the restoration of flow out of the portal vein by the stent can by itself efficiently treat

Figure 3.8
Treatment of recurrent encephalopathy after surgical mesentericocaval anastomosis (11 during the last 12 months). (a) Portography performed before TIPS placement, via a jugular route, shows a patent mesentericocaval shunt with a complete portal flow derivation to the inferior vena cava (IVC) (arrowheads). (b) After 14 months, encephalopathy was no longer observed and an angiogram demonstrated that the TIPS was patent (arrowheads) and the surgical shunt occluded by a detachable balloon (arrowheads).

(a)

(b)

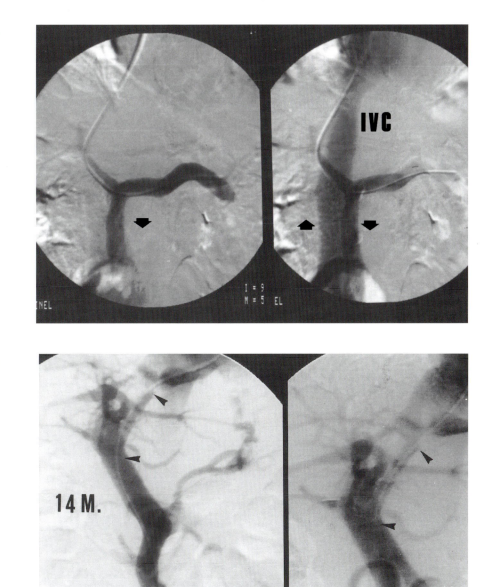

the portal thrombosis (Fig. 3.9). However, this treatment is less effective in the presence of cavernous transformation of the portal vein. Similarly, if the stent is placed too distally in a portal vein in a patient who is about to undergo a liver transplantation, surgical difficulties can be encountered because of difficulty of removal of the distally placed stent.

Encephalopathy is not an absolute contraindication. Indeed, encephalopathy occurring in the course of an acute bleeding episode is often transient and frequently regresses once the bleeding has stopped.

(a)

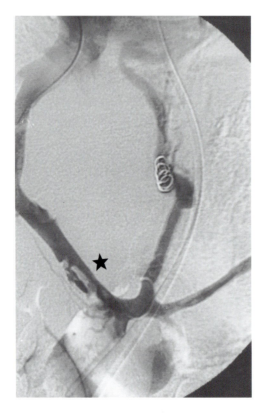

(b)

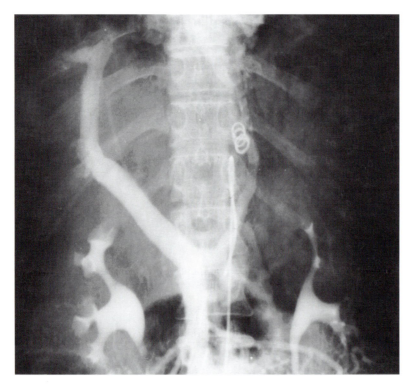

Figure 3.9
(a) TIPS performed in spite of a partial portal thrombosis (star) secondary to 2 thrombosed surgical portocaval anastomoses. (b) Angiographic control 1 year later showing patent TIPS with no residual thrombi in portal vein.

Comments

Despite the great advances reported in the performance of the TIPS procedure during the last few years, a number of unanswered questions remain, the first of which relates to the exact role of this procedure in comparison with other methods of treatment of portal hypertension. TIPS has proved efficacious in treating patients with haemorrhage refractory to medical treatment; however, the results are awaited of large, controlled prospective studies comparing the efficacy of TIPS with other therapeutic methods in preventing recurrent haemorrhage in patients with liver cirrhosis.

Can this technique be applied universally? Sclerotherapy is a relatively easy-to-learn procedure and can be performed in routine clinical practice, even in a small hospital. On the other hand, the performance of TIPS requires an experienced interventional radiologist and associated radiologic personnel who are trained to perform the procedure, have the appropriate equipment necessary, and are willing to commit themselves to the treatment of these patients.

What is the ideal shunt diameter? Normalizing the portosystemic pressure gradient exposes the patient to the combined risk of encephalopathy and progressive deterioration of hepatic function. According to published data, a portacaval pressure gradient below 12 mmHg is sufficient for protection from haemorrhagic risk.[69,70] However, although portal pressure should be sufficiently reduced to prevent haemorrhage, complete normalization can lead to encephalopathy. According to Poiseuille's law, resistance in a vessel and resistance in a tube are inversely proportional to the 4th power of the radius. Therefore, very small variations in shunt calibre have important repercussions on resistance to intra-anastomotic flow. Thus, the flow obtained with one 12 mm stent is equivalent to the flow obtained with two 10 mm stents. The placement of large stents that can result in excessive decrease of portal pressure should be avoided. Nevertheless, it is known that, during the months following a stent placement, a physiological narrowing of the shunt secondary to intimal hyperplasia will occur. Consequently, a 10 mm shunt will decrease in size to approximately 8 mm 4 months later. Should shunts, therefore, be equal; should they actually be calibrated to a greater size than desired at initial implantation because it is known that they will shrink because of intimal hyperplasia? These are difficult questions to answer and at this point it is necessary to compromise between the risk of recurrent haemorrhage and encephalopathy.

The major limitation of the TIPS procedure is intimal hyperplasia. It increases with time and requires frequent reinterventions. At present, there are no specific methods for the treatment of this complication. Anticoagulants have not proved effective, and haemorrhagic complications with the use of anticoagulants create a risk greater than the expected benefit.

The answer to the problem of shunt obstruction may lie in the development of covered shunts, which would avoid biliary fistulae and intimal proliferation. The authors have performed experimental animal trials using a Dacron-coated Cragg shunt, which demonstrated a 70% secondary occlusion rate. This could be due to the characteristic properties of Dacron, which has been shown in vascular surgical studies not to function well in small-diameter bypasses.[72] Early experimental work by Nishimine *et al.* with poly(tetrafluoroethene)-covered prostheses seems to have demonstrated longer patency.[73] However, this type of prosthesis is technically difficult to implant, and is still associated with a small incidence of intimal hyperplasia.

In conclusion, over the past few years TIPS has proved to be a feasible and relatively safe technique. Results suggest that it is helpful in treatment of uncontrolled or refractory haemorrhage in patients in whom other methods of treatment have failed. It also seems to be of some use in patients with refractory ascites. However, long-term patency is not possible and close surveillance and frequent reinterventions should be expected.

References

1   Ready JB, Rector WG. Morbidity and mortality of portal hypertension. *Drugs* 1989; **37**(Suppl. 2): 13–24.

2   Pagliaro L, Burroughs AK, Sorensen TIA *et al.* Therapeutic controversies and randomised controlled trials (RCTs): Prevention of bleeding and rebleeding in cirrhosis. *Gastroenterol Int* 1989; **2**: 71–84.

3   Terblanche J, Burroughs AK, Hobbs KEF. Controversies in the management of bleeding oesophageal varices. *N Engl J Med* 1989; **320**: 1469–1475.

4   Teres J, Bordas JM, Bravo D *et al.* Sclerotherapy versus distal spleno renal shunt in the elective treatment of variceal hemorrhage: a randomized controlled trial. *Hepatology* 1987; **7**: 430–436.

5   Cello JP, Grendell JP, Crass RA, Weber TE, Trunkey DD. Endoscopic sclerotherapy versus portacaval shunt in patients with severe cirrhosis and acute variceal hemorrhage. *N Engl J Med* 1987; **316**: 11–15.

6   Rösch J, Hanafee W, Snow H. Transjugular portal venography and radiologic portacaval shunt: an experimental study. *Radiology* 1969; **92**: 1112–1114.

7   Rösch J, Hanafee W, Snow H, Barenfus M, Gray R. Transjugular intrahepatic portacaval shunt. *Am J Surg* 1971; **121**: 588–592.

8   Rösch J. Non surgical intrahepatic portacaval shunt: a utopian dream or an approaching reality? *Hepatology* 1986; **6**(5): 1056–1058.

9   Palmaz JC, Sibbit RR, Reuter SR, Garcia F, Tio FO. Expandable intrahepatic portacaval shunts stents: early experience in the dog. *AJR* 1985; **145**: 821–825.

10   Rösch J, Uchida BT, Putnam JS, Buschman RW, Law RD, Hershey AL. Experimental intrahepatic portacaval anastomosis: use of expandable Gianturco stents. *Radiology* 1987; **162**: 481–485.

11   Palmaz JC, Garcia F, Sibbit RR. Expandable intrahepatic portacaval shunt stents in dogs with chronic portal hypertension. *AJR* 1986; **147**: 1251–1254.

12   Rousseau H, Bilbao I, Vinel JP, Maquin P, Longo J, Joffre F. Experimental porto hepatic shunt with the Wallstent endoprostheses. *SCVIR*, San Francisco 16–21 Feb 1991 (abstract).

13   Richter GM, Palmaz JC, Noldge G *et al.* Der transjuguläre intrahepatische protosystemische stent-shunt (TIPSS). *Radiologe* 1989; **29**: 406–411.

14   Laberge JM, Ring EJ, Gordon RL *et al.* Creation of transjugular intrahepatic portosystemic shunts with Wallstent endoprosthesis: results in 100 patients. *Radiology* 1993; **187**: 413–420.

15   Richter GM, Noldge G, Rossle M, Palmaz JC. Evolution and clinical introduction of TIPSS, the transjugular intrahepatic portosystemic stent-shunt. *Semin Intervent Radiol* 1991; **8** 231–240.

16   Zemel G, Katzen BT, Becker GJ, Benenati JF, Sallee S. Percutaneous transjugular portosystemic shunt. *JAMA* 1991; **266**: 390–393.

17   Rousseau H, Vinel JP, Bilbao I, Longo J, Zozaya JM, Maquin P. Transjugular intra hepatic portosystemic shunts using the Wallstent endoprosthesis: a follow-up study. *Cardiovasc Intervent Radiol* 1994; **17**: 7–11.

18   Laberge JM, Ring EJ, Gordon RL. Percutaneous intrahepatic portosystemic shunt created via a femoral vein approach. *Radiology* 1991; **181**: 679–681.

19   Longo JM, Bilbao JI, Rousseau HP *et al.* Color doppler US guidance in transjugular placement of intrahepatic portosystemic shunts. *Radiology* 1992; **184**: 281–284.

20   Teisseire R, Clanet J, Broussy P, Cassigneul J, Fourtanier G, Pascal JP. Abord transjugulaire du système porte. Applications au diagnostic, au pronostic et à la thérapeutique des hémorragies digestives du cirrhotique. *Gastroenterol Clin Biol* 1979; **3**: 425–432.

21   Colapinto RF, Stronell RD, Gildiner M. Formation of intrahepatic portosystemic shunts using a balloon dilatation catheter: preliminary clinical experience. *AJR* 1983; **140**: 709–714.

22   Echenagusia AJ, Camunez F, Simo G *et al.* Variceal hemorrhage: efficacy of transjugular intrahepatic portosystemic shunts created with Strecker stents. *Radiology* 1994; **192**: 235–240.

23   Longo J, Bilbao J, Rousseau H *et al.* Transjugular intrahepatic portosystemic shunt evaluation with Doppler sonography. *Radiology* 1993; **186**: 529–584.

24 Chong WK, Malisch TA, Mazer MJ, Lind CD, Worrel JA, Richards WO. Transjugular intrahepatic portosystemic shunt: US assessment with maximum flow velocity. *Radiology* 1993; **189**: 789–793.

25 Feldstein V, Laberge J. Hepatic vein flow reversal at duplex sonography: a sign of transjugular intrahepatic portosystemic shunt dysfunction. *AJR* 1994; **162**: 839–841.

26 Sabba C, Weltin GG, Cicchetti DV *et al*. Observer variability in echo-Doppler measurements of portal flow in cirrhotic patients and normal volunteers. *Gastroenterology* 1990; **98**: 1603–1611.

27 Rossle M, Haag K, Hauenstein H *et al*. TIPS using Palmaz stent or Wallstent: randomized comparison of stenosis, occlusion, rebleeding and mortality (abstract). *J Hepatol* 1993; **18**(Suppl. 1): S165.

28 Keller FS, Rösch J. Results of TIPS (abstract). 2nd International Workshop on Interventional Radiology, Prague, 15–17 June 1995.

29 Rossle M, Haag K, Ochs A *et al*. The transjugular intrahepatic portosystemic stent-shunt procedure for variceal bleeding. *N Engl J Med* 1994; **330**: 165–171.

30 Helton W, Belshaw A, Althaus S *et al*. Critical appraisal of the angiographic portacaval shunt (TIPS). *Am J Surg* 1993; **165**: 566–571.

31 Perarnau J, Raabe J, Schwing D *et al*. Anastomose portocave intrahépatique par voie transjugulaire: résultats préliminaires. *Gastroenterol Clin Biol* 1993; **17**: 422–430.

32 Jalan R, Redhead D, Simpson K, Elton RA, Hayes PC. Transjugular intrahepatic portosystemic stent shunts (TIPSS): long term follow up. *Q J Med* 1994; **87**: 365–373.

33 Coldwell DM, Ring EJ, Rees CR *et al*. Multicenter investigation of the role of transjugular intrahepatic portosystemic shunt in management of portal hypertension. *Radiology* 1995; **196**: 335–340.

34 McCormick PA, Dick R, Panagou EB *et al*. Emergency transjugular intrahepatic portosystemic stent shunting as salvage treatment for uncontrolled variceal bleeding. *Br J Surg* 1994; **81**: 1324–1327.

35 Sanyal A, Freedman A, Purdum P *et al*. Transjugular intrahepatic portosystemic shunting (TIPS) versus sclerotherapy for prevention of recurrent variceal hemorrhage: a randomized prospective trial (abstract). *Gastroenterology* 1994; **106**: A975.

36 Rossle M, Deibert P, Hagg K, Ochs A, Siegerstetter V, Langer M. TIPS vs sclerotherapy and beta blockade: preliminary results of a randomized study in patients with recurrent hemorrhage (abstract). *Hepatology* 1994; **20**: 44.

37 Cabrera J, Maynar M, Granados R *et al*. TIPS vs sclerotherapy in the elective treatment of variceal bleeding: a randomized control study (abstract). *Hepatology* 1994; **20**: 425.

38 Vinel JP, Rousseau H and Groupe d'étude des anastomoses intrahépatiques (France). TIPS vs sclerotherapy + propranolol in the prevention of variceal bleeding: preliminary results of a multicenter randomized trial (abstract). Hepatology 1995; (in press).

39 Bezzi M, Merli M, Riggio O, Salvatori FM, Capocaccia L, Rossi M, Rossi P. Transjugular portosystemic shunt vs endoscopic sclerotherapy in the prevention of variceal bleeding: a randomized trial (abstract). CIRSE, *Cardiovasc Intervent Radiol* 1995; **10**(Suppl. 1) S 59.

40 Quiroga J, Sangro B, Nunez M *et al*. Transjugular intrahepatic portal-systemic shunt in the treatment of refractory ascites: effect on clinical, renal, humoral, and hemodynamic parameters. *Hepatology* 1995; **21**: 986–994.

41 Ochs A, Rossle M, Haag K *et al*. The transjugular intrahepatic portosystemic stent shunt: procedure for refractory ascites. *N Engl J Med* 1995; **332**: 1192–1197.

42 Wong F, Sniderman K, Liu P, Allidina Y, Sherman M, Blendis I. Transjugular intrahepatic portosystemic stent shunt: effects on hemodynamics and sodium homeostasis in cirrhosis and refractory ascites. *Ann Intern Med* 1995; **122**: 816–822.

43 Somberg KA, Lake JR, Tomlanovich SJ, Laberge JM, Feldstein V Bass NM. Transjugular intrahepatic portosystemic shunts for refractory ascites: assessment of clinical and hormonal response and renal function. *Hepatology* 1995; **21**: 709–716.

44 Gines P, Arroyo V, Vargas V *et al*. Paracentesis with intravenous infusion of albumin as compared with peritoneovenous shunting in cirrhosis with refractory ascites. *N Engl J Med* 1991; **325**: 829–835.

45 Lebrec D, Giuily N, Hadengue A *et al*. Transjugular intrahepatic portosystemic shunt (TIPS) vs paracentesis for refractory ascites. Results of a randomized trial (abstract). *Hepatology* 1994; **20**: 201 A.

46 Laberge JM, Somberg KA, Lake JR *et al*. Two-year outcome following transjugular intrahepatic portosystemic shunt for variceal bleeding: results in 90 patients. *Gastroenterology* 1995; **108**: 1142–1151.

47 Rubin RA, Haskal ZJ, O'Brien CB, Cope C, Brass CA. Transjugular intrahepatic portosystemic shunting: decreased survival for patients with high Apache II scores. *Am J Gastroenterol* 1995; **90**(4): 556–563.

48 Pattynama PMT, Van Hoek B, Kool LJ. Inadvertent arteriovenous stenting during transjugular intrahepatic portosystemic shunt procedure and the importance of hepatic artery perfusion. *Cardiovasc Intervent Radiol* 1995; **18**: 192–195.

49 Haskal ZJ, Pentecost MJ, Rubin A. Hepatic arterial injury after transjugular intrahepatic portosystemic shunt placement: report of two cases. *Radiology* 1993; **188**: 85–88.

50 Sanyal AJ, Freedman AM, Purdum PP. TIPS associated hemolysis and encephalopathy. *Ann Intern Med* 1992; **117**: 443–444.

51 Freedman A, Sanyal A, Tisnado J *et al*. Complications of transjugular intrahepatic portosystemic shunt: a comprehensive review. *Radiographics* 1993; **13**: 1185–1210.

52 Azoulay D, Castaing D, Dennison A, Martino W, Eyraud D, Bismuth H. Transjugular intrahepatic portosystemic shunt worsens the hyperdynamic circulatory state of the cirrhotic patient: preliminary report of a prospective study. *Hepatology* 1994; **19**: 129–132.

53 Sellinger M, Ochs A, Haag K. Incidence of hepatic encephalopathy and follow-up of liver function in patients with transjugular intrahepatic portosystemic stent-shunt (TIPS) (abstract). *Gastroenterology* 1992; **102**: A 883.

54 Somberg KA, Riegler JL, Doherty M *et al*. Hepatic encephalopathy following transjugular intrahepatic portosystemic shunts (TIPS): incidence and risk factors (abstract). *Hepatology* 1992; **16**(Suppl.): 122 A.

55 Sanyal AJ, Freedman AM, Shiffman ML *et al*. Portosystemic encephalopathy after transjugular intrahepatic portosystemic shunt: results of a prospective controlled study. *Hepatology* 1994; **20**: 46–55.

56 Nazarian GK, Ferral H, Castaneda–Zuniga WR *et al*. Development of stenoses in transjugular intrahepatic portosystemic shunts. *Radiology* 1994; **192**: 231–234.

57 Hausegger KA, Sternthal HM, Klein GE, Karaic R, Stauber R, Zenker G. Transjugular intrahepatic portosystemic shunt: angiographic follow-up and secondary interventions. *Radiology* 1994; **191**: 177–181.

58 Haskal Z , Pentecost M, Soulen M *et al*. Transjugular intrahepatic portosystemic shunt stenosis and revision: early and midterm results. *AJR* 1994; **163**: 439–444.

59 Theilmann I, Sauer P, Roeren T *et al*. Acetylsalicylic acid in the prevention of early stenosis and occlusion of transjugular intrahepatic portal-systemic stent shunts: a controlled study. *Hepatology* 1994; **20**: 592–597.

60 Jalan R, Harrison D, Redhead D *et al*. The role of transient biliary venous fistula in the pathogenesis of shunt occlusion following TIPSS (abstract). *Hepatology* 1994; **20**: 103A.

61 Vinel JP, Rousseau H. Transjugular intrahepatic portosystemic shunts using the Wallstent endoprothesis: histological study in animals and in patients. *J Hepatol* 1992; **16**(Suppl. 1): S9 (abstract).

62 Ring EJ, Lake JR, Roberts JP *et al*. Using transjugular intrahepatic portosystemic shunts to control variceal bleeding before liver transplantation. *Ann Intern Med* 1992; **116**: 304–309.

63 Kuradusenge PH, Rousseau H, Vinel JP *et al*. Traitement des hemorragies par rupture de varices cardiotubérositaires par anastomose portosystemique intrahepatique par voie transjugulaire. *Gastroenterol Clin Biol* 1993; **17**: 431–434.

64 Moulin G, Champsaur P, Bartoli JM, Chagnaud C, Rousseau H, Monges D. TIPS for portal decompression to allow palliative treatment of adenocarcinoma of the oesophagus. *Cardiovasc Intervent Radiol* 1995; **18**: 186–188.

65 Peltzer MY, Ring EJ, Laberge JM, Haskal ZJ, Radosevitch PM, Gordon RL. Treatments of Budd–Chiari syndrome with a transjugular intrahepatic portosystemic shunt. *J Vasc Intervent Radiol* 1993; **4**: 263–267.

66 Walker HS, Rholl KS, Register TE, Van Breda A. Percutaneous placement of a hepatic vein stent in the treatment of Budd–Chiari syndrome. *J Vasc Intervent Radiol* 1990; **1**: 23–27.

67 Fujimoto M, Moriyasu F, Someda H, Kajimura K *et al*. Budd–Chiari syndrome: recanalization of an occluded hepatic vein with percutaneous transluminal angioplasty and a metallic stent. *J Vasc Intervent Radiol* 1993; **4**: 257–261.

68 Strauss R, Martin L, Kaufmann S *et al*. TIPS for the management of symptomatic cirrhotic hydrothorax. *Am J Gastroenterol* 1994; **89**: 1520–1522.

69 Rikkers IF, Sorrel WT, Jin G. Which portosystemic shunt is best? *Gastroenterol Clin North Am* 1992; **21**: 179–196.

70 Rypins EB, Sarfeh IJ. Does portal pressure influence direction of portal flow and encephalopathy rates after 10 mm portacaval shunts in man? *J Surg Res* 1984; **37**: 119–122.

71 Feu F, Cirera I, Garcia-Pagan JC *et al*. Portal pressure response to drug therapy predicts the risk of rebleeding from esophageal varices (abstract). *J Hepatol* 1992; **16**(Suppl. 1): S 37.

72 Otal P, Rousseau H, Vinel JP, Joffre D, Ducuin H, Pieraggi MT. TIPS with covered stents: results of an experimental study. (abstr S 12). *Cardiovasc Intervent Radiol* 1995, **18**(Suppl. 1)

73 Nishimine K, Saxon RR, Kichikiwa K. Improved transjugular intrahepatic portosystemic shunt patency with PTFE-covered stent-grafts: experimental results in swine. *Radiology* 1995; **196**: 341–347.

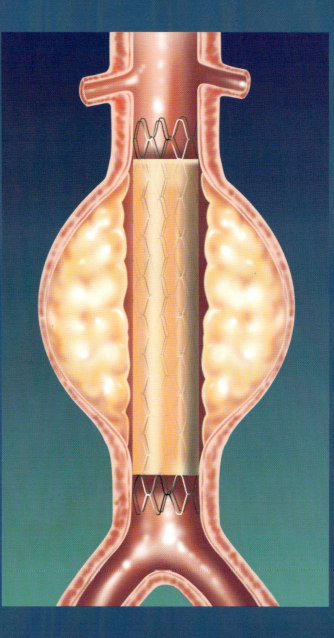

Chapter 4

Current status of endovascular stent grafts: an overview of applications and devices

B.T. Katzen

Introduction

During the past several years there has been increasing interest and investigation in the use of stent grafts to treat aneurysms and other vascular disorders. This has resulted from initial attempts to expand stent technology to more innovative approaches.[1] The purpose of this chapter is to provide an overview of a variety of approaches to developing endovascular stent grafts, give some insight into a rapidly developing field, and report initial experience in utilizing stent grafts at the Miami Vascular Institute.

Basic principles

The term 'stent graft' describes a device that integrates stents or stent-like devices with graft material to form a device that has functional properties greater than either a stent or graft alone. In the case of stents, these additional properties would include an impervious barrier, added length and, perhaps, flexibility, whereas grafts might have added support and the ability to be placed and fixed in place without surgical anastomosis. In this rapidly developing area other terms including 'stented grafts' and 'endovascular grafts' have also been suggested.[2] Undoubtedly, the terminology will evolve in conjunction with technological advances to accurately reflect the nature of devices.

Potential applications for this technology include the treatment of atherosclerotic aneurysms of the abdominal aorta and peripheral vessels, traumatic arteriovenous fistulae and aneurysms, and treatment of atherosclerotic occlusive disease. Functional specifications for an optimal device will vary depending on the pathology and anatomical region.

A variety of stent grafts are under investigation and, for simplicity, can best be described by their construction. All attempt to provide a luminal surface more impervious than stents alone, and to be placed in a less invasive manner than traditional bypass grafts. For purposes of discussion, stent grafts may conveniently be characterized as follows.

Covered stents

Perhaps the simplest form of stented graft may be created by applying a covering of graft material to a balloon-expandable or self-expanding stent. This type was employed in the first reported clinical use of an endovascular graft.[3] Examples include Gianturco™ Z-stents (Cook, Inc., Bloomington, IN)[4] covered with polyester, the covering of balloon-expandable Palmaz™ (Johnson & Johnson Interventional Systems, NJ) stents with polytetrafluoroethene (PTFE) and the use of nitinol covered with polyester (Endopro, MinTec, Freeport, Bahamas) for treatment of large aneurysms and occlusive disease. Only the Endopro is being manufactured and evaluated in clinical trials (in Europe); the others have been evaluated by individual investigators without industry participation.

Stents used for 'anastomosis' or attachment mechanism

Balloon-expandable stents have been used as anchoring mechanisms for graft material sewn to the stent prior to deployment. This method has been described and widely used by Parodi[5] for the treatment of aneurysms, and by others for the treatment of occlusive disease.[6] Others have utilized self-expanding 'attachment' mechanisms for anchoring the indwelling graft. These include a tube and bifurcated device being evaluated by Endovascular Technologies (Menlo Park, CA) Endovascular Grafting System,[7] and investigational efforts described by Chuter et al.[8]

Integrated weaves

Several types of vascular stents are manufactured using industrial weaving or knitting technology, including the Strecker stent, utilizing a balloon-expandable 'co-knit' of tantalum and polyester (Boston Scientific Corporation, Watertown, MA)[9] and a self-expanding device manufactured by Corvita Corporation (Miami, FL) both in early clinical trials in Europe. Advantages of this type of stent graft include reduced delivery size and flexibility, facilitating delivery in tortuous vessels.

Method of deployment

Devices may be further characterized by their method of deployment, either balloon-expandable or self-expandable. Some self-expanding types may still require use of compliant balloons to facilitate full expansion or attachment to the vessel wall.

Clinical applications

Several potential applications for stent grafts have been identified; however, these devices offer a unique opportunity for the treatment of aneurysms, particularly in the abdominal aorta and other large arteries. Naturally, the specifications and physical characteristics of endografts will vary depending on the clinical application. Applications being explored by various investigators include:

- abdominal aortic aneurysms
- thoracic aneurysms

- peripheral aneurysms
- peripheral arterial dissections
- arteriovenous fistulae
- aorto-iliac occlusive disease
- infra-inguinal occlusive disease
- traumatic arterial lesions.

Abdominal aortic aneurysms

Abdominal aortic aneurysms (AAAs) are most often asymptomatic and are discovered incidentally during radiographic or ultrasound examination of the abdomen for other reasons. While their natural history and prevalence is not entirely understood, studies have shown that progressive enlargement will occur in most patients, and that an individual's risk of rupture seems to be associated with aneurysm size.[10] While the mortality rate for rupture of these aneurysms is as high as 70%, elective repair of the aneurysm is associated with relatively low mortality and morbidity rates of 5% in most series. The risk of rupture and combined risks from surgery are approximately equal in aneurysms of 5 cm;[11] this is the basis for the prevailing opinion that these aneurysms should be operated on when reaching 5 cm, unless associated medical risk factors preclude therapy.

Recently, several devices have been developed for treating AAAs via endovascular techniques. While this is an extremely active area of investigation, and no approved devices are available for therapy in the United States, the following reviews attempt to address the present state of investigation.

Endovascular Technologies' Endovascular Grafting System

The EVT Endovascular Grafting System (EGS; Endovascular Technologies, Menlo Park, CA) consists of both a delivery system and endograft. A multicentre trial is currently under way in the United States to evaluate the safety and efficacy of this device for elective treatment of AAAs under an FDA Investigational Device Exemption (IDE). The trial began with a limited, phase I trial and, after clinical success, a phase II prospective randomized trial is currently under way. The trial is designed to compare the safety and efficacy of this device with conventional surgery.

The graft segment is made of woven polyester with self-expanding zigzag attachments sutured to each end of the tube graft (Fig. 4.1). Radio-opaque markers are sutured along the sides of the graft segment to facilitate fluoroscopic orientation and prevent rotation or twisting of the endograft. Graft diameter varies from 19 to 28 mm and length from 9.5 to 11 cm. The endograft is preloaded in a delivery system which is 24 Fr in size.

The device is placed via femoral artery cut-down, utilizing fluoroscopic localization, and a positioning device is placed under the patient prior to the procedure, which allows the interventionist to establish a fixed, radio-opaque landmark for use during deployment. The specifics of technique are beyond the scope of this discussion; however a variety of manoeuvres are required to allow precise deployment.

Patient selection includes those who would be considered candidates for conventional surgery, and have anatomical features of the aneurysm suitable for the device. These include well-defined proximal and distal necks of sufficient

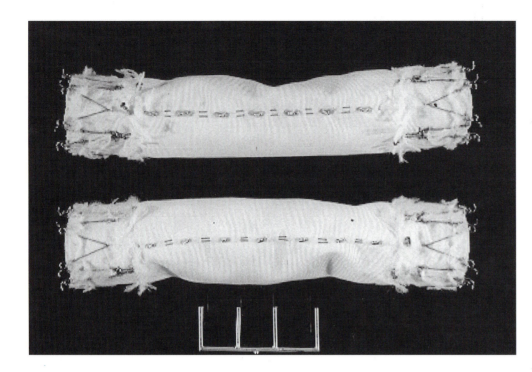

Figure 4.1
Endovascular Technologies Tube graft. Note self-expanding attachment mechanism with hooks for fixation. Radio-opaque markers are along the side of the endograft. Tufts of material at ends promote sealing.

length to allow seating of the attachment mechanism (15 mm length). Extreme angulation of the proximal neck will preclude patient inclusion. Additionally, patients must have iliac arteries of size and configuration suitable for introduction of the delivery mechanism.

Initial experience[12] has shown that this device can effectively isolate AAAs in certain patients (Fig. 4.2). With the delivery system being evaluated in the trial, successful implantation resulted in 94% of patients, with the need to convert to open surgery occurring in 6% of patients. Persistent filling of the aneurysm sac from either distal leaks or persistently patent lumbar arteries has been observed. Most leaks that are noted angiographically at the time of deployment have been found to close spontaneously during follow-up, but some have persisted into long-term follow-up. In one patient there was minimal enlargement of the AAA and surgical repair of the distal attachment was performed uneventfully. Complete understanding of the efficacy of this device will not be possible until the trial is complete.

Recently, a phase I trial of a bifurcated device was undertaken with successful implantation in 9 out of 11 patients. This device is not limited by the absence of a distal neck, but could still be limited by severe tortuosity of the proximal neck or the proximal iliac arteries.

Vanguard®

The Vanguard® (Meadox, Boston Scientific Corporation, Oakland, NJ, USA) (formerly Stentor®, Endotec/MinTec, Freeport, Bahamas) has been in clinical trials in several European centres. At the time of writing, a controlled prospective trial was not underway.

The Vanguard® is a nitinol, self-expanding device covered with Dacron sutured to the stent skeleton at various intervals. It is deployed through an 18 Fr

Figure 4.2
67-year-old with 5 cm saccular aneurysm of the abdominal aorta. (a) Angiogram prior to therapy. (b) Post EVT endograft placement. Note exclusion of aneurysm and attachment devices at proximal and distal neck.

(a)

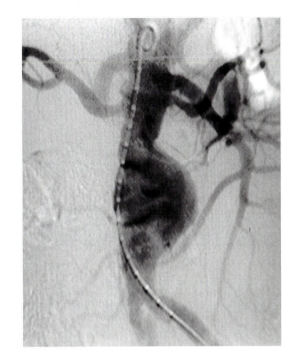

(b)

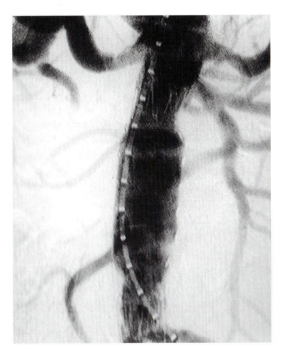

delivery system, which is placed through a femoral arteriotomy. The principal portion of the stent consists of an aortic limb and continuous iliac limb, with short contralateral cuff similar to a pair of trousers with one long and one short leg. The contralateral limb is then placed percutaneously from the contralateral iliac artery. Extensions can be placed if necessary.

Experience has been gained by several European investigators with a success rate in implantation of approximately 90%.[13] The device has been placed successfully in patients with an iliac artery aneurysm and no inferior aneurysm neck. Investigators have reported a 'post implant syndrome' in which pain and prolonged fever, without evidence of sepsis, has been documented. Elevated white blood cell count, C-reactive protein, and reduction in platelets has also been noted in patients receiving this device for the treatment of AAAs.

'Co-knit'

Some investigators have postulated that aneurysms might be excluded by placement of a device that is porous but induces thrombosis of the sac, and thereby protection from expansion and rupture. Experimental work utilizing Strecker stents demonstrated that, by reducing pore size, thrombosis could be induced in experimental models.

Utilizing industrial knitting methods, a stent-like device combining both metal (tantalum) and fabric (polyester), or so-called 'co-knit', is being evaluated in phase I clinical trials.[9] Advantages include reduced profile and size of introduction (14–16 Fr), flexibility, and component configuration allowing variability in deployment. With very limited clinical experience, successful deployment has been accomplished in all patients with no need for conversion to conventional surgery. Additionally, thrombosis of the AAA has been observed. In long-term follow-up, patency of the IMA and some lumbar arteries has been noted, similar to the way stents have preserved collateral vessels when placed across ostia. Further investigation will be required to address these poorly understood issues.

Covered JJIS stents

Similar, limited clinical investigation has been conducted with covered large balloon-expandable stents, utilizing a covering of PTFE sutured to a 50 mm extra-large stent deployed on a specially designed balloon catheter. In 8 patients, 6 devices were successfully placed with exclusion of the AAA.[14] A clinical trial is not yet under way. This type of approach using smaller stents is discussed further below.

Other applications for stent grafts

As mentioned above, other types of vascular pathology may benefit from evolving stent graft technology. Traumatic lesions may be managed by a variety of approaches including simple covered stents as described or with more complex endovascular procedures.[15] Additionally, pseudoaneurysms at anastomotic areas may also be treated by stent graft placement utilizing devices such as covered Palmaz stents (Fig. 4.3).[16] These types of devices can be manufactured in the angiography suite and are available for traumatic or other applications where a rigid balloon-expandable stent is needed. Obviously, in treating anastomotic breakdown, consideration should be given to the possibility of graft infection as the cause. Larger aneurysms such as those occurring in the thoracic aorta can be effectively treated using self-expanding Gianturco Z-stents covered with polyester (Fig. 4.4).[17] Peripheral aneurysms may also be treated with these devices or more simply with commercially available stents (in Europe) such as the Cragg Endopro (Fig. 4.5). Treatment of aortic dissections may be facilitated with endovascular stent grafts and the author's limited experience along with others[18] with Type B dissections seems to indicate a role which also has some experimental

Figure 4.3

68-year-old with severe left hip and thigh pain. (a) Spiral CT scan demonstrates large pelvic pseudoaneurysm. (b) Angiogram demonstrates 'jet' on contrast into pseudoaneurysm from anastomosis. Previous occlusion of right limb of aortobifemoral bypass graft. (c) Palmaz balloon-expandable stents covered with PTFE, one mounted and one unmounted. Note that the fabric is not sewn all the way to the ends of the stent due to foreshortening. (d) Angiogram following deployment of two covered stents shows exclusion of aneurysm.

(a)

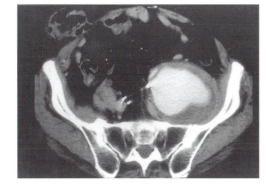

(b)

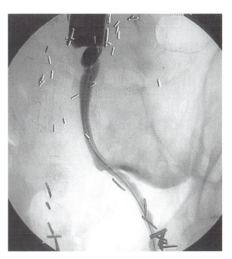

(c)

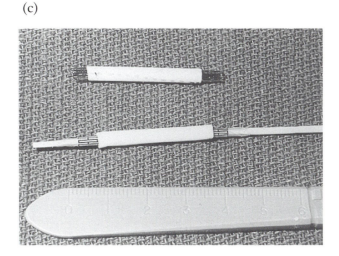

(d)

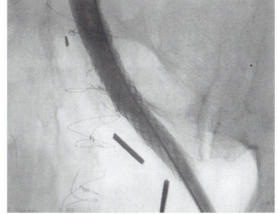

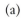

(a)

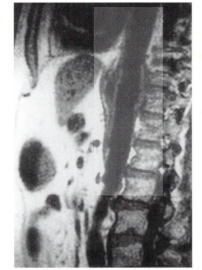

(b)

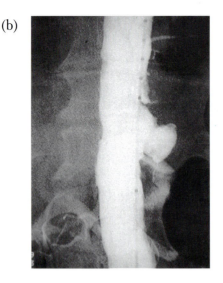

(c)

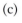

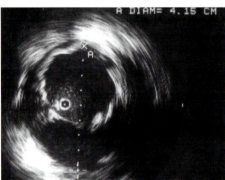

A DIAM= 4.15 CM

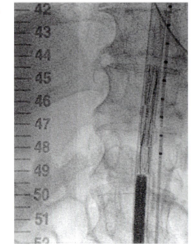

(d)

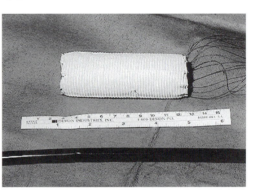

(e)

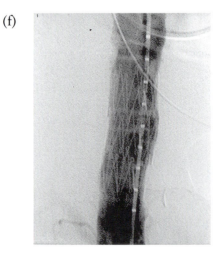

(f)

Figure 4.4
78-year-old woman with 6-week history of interscapular pain. (a) Lateral MR scan showing 'contained' rupture of lower thoracic aorta. (b) Thoracic angiogram demonstrating penetrating ulcer of distal thoracic aorta. (c) Intravascular ultrasound showing haematoma surrounding lumen. (d) Gianturco Z-Stent covered with polyester. Sutures at the end are to facilitate loading of this self-expanding device into a delivery capsule. (e) Radiograph of endograft in delivery sheath prior to deployment. (f) Completion angiogram showing exclusion of the diseased area.

Figure 4.5
Aneurysm of the right common iliac artery aneurysm in a patient with vague pelvic pain. (a) Pelvic angiogram: contrast filling portion of penetration right common iliac artery aneurysm. (b) Self-expanding nitinol stent covered with Dacron. (c) Completion angiogram showing successful exclusion of aneurysm. Hospital stay: 23 hours. (d) CT scan shows exclusion of iliac aneurysm.

(a)

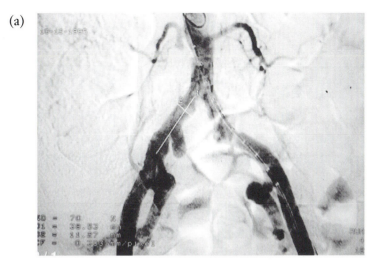

(b)

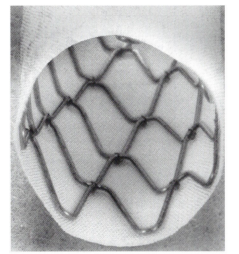

(c)

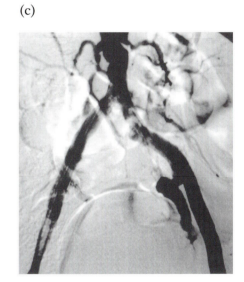

(d)

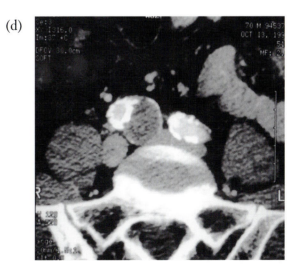

basis.[19] Another area of future development is in the endovascular treatment of occlusive disease. It is hoped that the use of materials will improve the initial and long-term success rates of interventional therapy, particularly in areas such as the superficial femoral artery. These are all areas for future investigation as experience is currently limited.

Characteristics of an optimal stent graft

For stent grafts to fulfil the potential advantages they offer when compared with conventional surgery, certain characteristics can be defined as desirable, and some even as critical. Some of these are identified below.

Device size. It would be most desirable for devices to have high expansion ratios allowing them to be introduced by relatively small (even percutaneous) methods. Delivery size should be as small as possible.

Biocompatibility. Materials used should have proven safety in human application since they will be permanently implanted. Durability should be proven.

Functionality. The device should either be impervious to blood or be capable of sealing within a short and reproducible period of time.

Flexibility. The device and delivery system should be able to negotiate the circulatory pathways necessary to deliver it to the site of therapy, such as tortuous iliac arteries, or the brachiocephalic vessels.

Predictable delivery system. Reproducible methods of delivery should exist, with few or no instances of device failure.

High radio-opacity. In the absence of surgical exposure, radio-opacity is critical to allow precise deployment. Certain types of devices might require additional markers to facilitate orientation, rotation and/or twisting.

Incorporate standard angiographic techniques. Accepted methods of catheterization ('over the wire') should be employed to facilitate delivery and reduce complications.

Rigidity. For use in occlusive disease, some rigidity and ability to resist elastic recoil is necessary. Similar functional specifications to those of uncovered intravascular stents.

Predictable and convenient sizing. This characteristic is particularly important in larger vessels, such as the thoracic aorta, in developing proper sealing of the proximal end of the stent graft, and in varying the iliac limbs for bifurcation disease.

Optimal environments for performing endovascular graft procedures

Endovascular grafts or stent grafts describe a diverse group of developing devices in varying sizes. Many can be delivered by percutaneous techniques, and some require surgical access. Both the technology and the clinical applications are evolving, raising questions about where the most optimal results can be obtained. Clearly, the procedures are imaging dependent and require interventional skills. Frequently, surgical skills are required to provide access and, in addition, patients may benefit from procedures combining both types of skill, for example endograft in one iliac artery followed by cross-femoral bypass. Many investigators are performing these types of procedures in the operating room environment; however, in the author's own institution, the potential of performing endovascular procedures in a slightly modified angiography suite has been evaluated.[20] In addition to percutaneous procedures, surgery ranging from arteriotomal to aortobifemoral bypass has been successfully performed, converting the interventional procedure to conventional surgery. In the author's preliminary experience of 34 patients there was an infection rate of 3.4%. The endovascular suite has been unanimously accepted by his surgical colleagues for a variety of procedures, and this alternative also has been used successfully by others.[21]

Conclusions

Endovascular grafts represent an exciting area of new development in vascular intervention. The ability to achieve endovascular exclusion of aneurysms and place synthetic grafts via endovascular approaches offers great promise and requires further investigation. Despite enthusiasm over initial results of this technology, appropriate caution should be exercised until some long-term benefit is achieved and proof of safety is established. Appropriate caution is warranted based on adverse events in a United States FDA Investigational Device Exemption study occurring despite abundant pre-investigation animal and 'bench top' testing.[22] Unanticipated longitudinal stress resulted in fractures in hooks on the attachment mechanism. After voluntary suspension of the clinical trial, significant improvements to the device led to a recent restart of the clinical trials of tube grafts, and phase I trial of a bifurcated device. Additionally, in some patients treated with a 'Parodi'-type device, delayed rupture of AAAs occurred resulting from continued expansion of the aneurysm neck proximal to the proximal anchoring stent leading to proximal leaks.[23] Although events of this type are bound to occur during the development and investigation of any new device, they emphasize the need for *cautious* optimism when evaluating and presenting new technology.

Certain types of devices may be of value to the interventionalist and patient in contemporary practice, including covered stents, some of which are available for clinical application in Europe, Asia and South America. Alternatively, utilizing materials available in the angiography and surgical environments, the interventionalist can fashion devices that can be introduced percutaneously and bring immediate patient benefit, avoiding more extensive surgery, particularly in cases of trauma, or peripheral aneurysm in patients who are poor surgical candidates.

The development and investigation of stent grafts is in its embryonic stages, and there is great promise for significant innovation in treatment of peripheral vascular occlusive and aneurysmal disease. Applications will be increasing as technology continues to improve.

References

1   Palmaz JC, Sibbitt RR, Reuter SR, Tio FO, Rice WJ. Expandable intraluminal graft: a feasibility study. Work in progress. *Radiology* 1985; **156**(1): 73–77.

2   Veith FJ, Abbott WM, Yao JS *et al*. Guidelines for development and use of transluminally placed endovascular prosthetic grafts in the arterial system. Endovascular Graft Committee. *J Vasc Surg* 1995; **21**(4): 670–685.

3   Becker GJ, Benenati JF, Zemel G *et al*. Percutaneous placement of a balloon-expandable intraluminal graft for life-threatening subclavian artery hemorrhage. *J Vasc Intervent Radiol* 1991; **2**: 225–229.

4   Dake MD, Miller DC, Semba CP, Mitchell RS, Walker PJ, Liddell RP. Transluminal placement of endovascular stent-grafts for the treatment of descending thoracic aortic aneurysms. *N Engl J Med* 1994; **331**(26): 1729–1734.

5   Parodi JC. Endovascular repair of abdominal aortic aneurysms and other arterial lesions. *J Vasc Surg* 1995; **21**(4): 549–555.

6   Cragg AH, Dake MD. Percutaneous femoropopliteal graft placement. *J Vasc Intervent Radiol* 1993; **4**(4): 455–463.

7   Lazarus HM. Endovascular grafting for the treatment of abdominal aortic aneurysms. *Surg Clin North Am* 1992; **72**: 959–968.

8   Chuter TA, Donayre C, Wendt G. Bifurcated stent-grafts for endovascular repair of abdominal aortic aneurysms: Preliminary case reports. *Surg Endosc* 1994; **8**(7): 800–802.

9   Picquet P, Rolland PH, Bartoli JM, Tranier P, Moulin G, Mercier C. Tantalum–Dacron co-knit stent for endovascular treatment of aortic aneurysms: a preliminary experimental study. *J Vasc Surg* 1994; **19**(4): 698–706.

10 Thurmond AS, Semler HJ. Abdominal aortic aneurysm: incidence in a population at risk. *J Cardiovasc Surg* 1986; **27**(4): 457.

11 Taylor LM, Proter JM. Basic data related to clinical decision making in abdominal aortic aneurysm. *Ann Vasc Surg* 1986; **1**: 500.

12 Moore WS, Rutherford RB for the EVT Investigators. Transfemoral endovascular repair of abdominal aortic aneurysm: results of the North American EVT phase I trial. *J Vasc Surg* 1996; **23**: 543–553.

13 Blum U, Steltor H. Paper presented at the 8th International Symposium on Vascular Diagnosis and Intervention. Miami, FL. January 28, 1996.

14 Richter GH. Paper presented at the 8th International Symposium on Vascular Diagnosis and Intervention. Miami, FL. January 28, 1996.

15 Marin ML, Veith FJ, Panetta TF *et al*. Transluminally placed endovascular stented graft repair for arterial trauma. *J Vasc Surg* 1994; **20**(3): 466–472.

16 Terry PJ, Houser EE, Rivera FJ, Palmaz JC, Sarosdy MF. Percutaneous aortic stent placement for life-threatening aortic rupture due to metastatic germ cell tumor. *J Urol* 1995; **153**(5): 1631–1634.

17 Lawrence DD Jr, Charnsangavej C, Wright KC, Gianturco C, Wallace S. Percutaneous endovascular graft: experimental evaluation. *Radiology* 1987; **163**(2): 357–360.

18 Walker PJ, Dake MD, Mitchell RS, Miller DC. The use of endovascular techniques for the treatment of complications of aortic dissection. *J Vasc Surg* 1993; **18**(6): 1042–1051.

19 Marty-Ane C, Serres-Cousine O, Laborde JC, Costes V, Alauzen M, Mary H. Use of endovascular stents for acute aortic dissection: an experimental study. *Ann Vasc Surg* 1994; **8**(5): 434–442.

20 Katzen BT, Becker GJ, Mascioli CA *et al*. Creation of a modified angiography (endovascular) suite for transluminally placed endograft placement and combined interventional–surgical procedures. *J Vasc Intervent Radiol* 1996; **7**: 161–167.

21 Blum U. Paper presented at the 8th International Symposium of Vascular Diagnosis and Intervention. Miami, FL. January 28, 1996.

22 Bernhardt V. Endovascular Technologies, Inc. Personal Communication. January 1995.

23 Parodi JC. Personal Communication. March 1996.

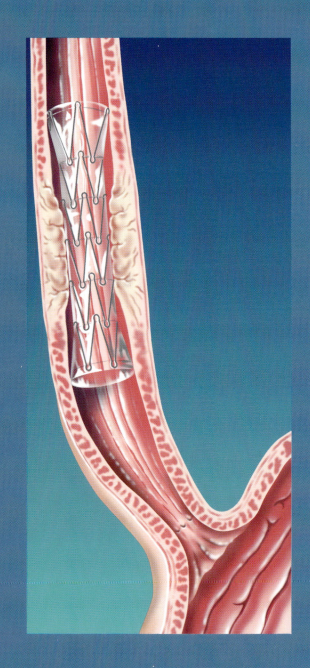

Chapter 5

Oesophageal stents

A.F. Watkinson, R.C. Mason and A. Adam

Introduction

The relatively recent introduction of self-expanding metallic endoprostheses for use in the treatment of oesophageal strictures has changed the approach to the management of what in many instances is a difficult clinical problem. In the treatment of benign disease, balloon dilatation remains the mainstay of treatment and metallic stents should be used as a last resort after detailed discussion with clinical colleagues.[1] In the palliation of inoperable malignant oesophageal obstruction, metallic stents are already making a significant contribution.

Oesophageal carcinoma is a relatively common disease, with an incidence of approximately 7.5 per 100,000 of the population. In more than 50% of patients curative resection is inappropriate and only palliative therapy is possible.[2] Traditional methods have included surgery,[3] radiotherapy[4,5] and plastic endoprostheses.[6–8]

Radiotherapy achieves an acceptable degree of palliation of dysphagia in approximately 40% of cases but it may take 2 months or longer to achieve its results. Plastic endoprostheses are inexpensive but have many limitations. Although the outer diameter of rigid plastic tubes is relatively large, and in most cases general anaesthesia is required for insertion, the lumen is relatively small and food impaction is frequent; most patients cannot eat solid food. Insertion of plastic tubes is associated with a mortality of up to 16% and with a dislodgement rate of approximately 20%. The overall complication rate is variable, but has been reported to be as high as 36–40%.[8]

Laser therapy[9–12] has been shown to be effective in relieving symptoms. The laser energy is administered via a flexible quartz fibre down the biopsy channel of an endoscope in a retrograde fashion. In a third of cases laser therapy requires pretreatment oesophageal dilatation, to enable the endoscope to pass into the stomach. Although this will enable over 80% of patients to swallow a semisolid diet, or better, treatment needs to be repeated on a 4 to 8-weekly basis. The morbidity and mortality are low (<5%) and are mainly related to perforation of the oesophagus during the pretreatment dilatation. Perforation is associated with a 13% mortality despite intensive medical therapy.[13] Trials comparing laser with conventional plastic endoprostheses demonstrate that laser produces better swallowing and is safer, but often requires a repeat procedure. In contrast, plastic tubes are cheaper and can be inserted in a one-off procedure, but patients usually manage only a liquid diet.[7]

Self-expanding metallic endoprostheses consist of a metal mesh, which may be uncovered or covered with some form of plastic in order to prevent ingrowth of tumour.[14–20] Metallic stents can be inserted under sedation using fluoroscopy alone in a 30–45-minute procedure, with relatively low morbidity and mortality.

Stent designs

Several types of self-expanding endoprostheses are available. The basic principle underlying their use is the same: an expansile tube of metal mesh is compressed and then inserted while restrained on a delivery device of small diameter. When the stent is positioned in the stricture the restraining device is removed and the mesh expands against the stricture. Insertion can be performed under sedation using standard X-ray equipment. As metallic stents expand to a large diameter, they achieve excellent palliation of dysphagia. Several studies have shown that the technical success rate of satisfactory insertion of these devices approaches 100%,[14–18] with very good palliation of symptoms. However, a proportion of them become occluded due to ingrowth of tumour through the metallic mesh.[16] In view of this, new stent designs have been produced, which are covered with some form of plastic such as polyethylene or polyurethane, in order to prevent tumour growing through the mesh.[15,17,18]

The main types of metallic endoprostheses available today are the Ultraflex device (Boston Scientific, Medi-tech Inc., Watertown, MA 02172, USA), the Gianturco stent (William Cook Europe, A/S Bjaeverskov, Denmark) and the Wallstent™ endoprosthesis (Schneider AG, Bulach, Switzerland).[15–18]

Ultraflex device (Figure 5.1)

This is a knitted mesh of 0.15 inch nitinol wire which is a self-expanding metallic alloy of nickel and titanium. This device is flexible in both the radial and the longitudinal axes. It has a maximum expanded outer diameter of 18 mm and is available in lengths of 7, 10 and 15 cm. The proximal end of the stent is amplified into a 5-mm long collar with a diameter of 20 mm. The mesh is compressed into an 8 mm diameter delivery system with a 60-cm long covering Teflon sheath. The mesh is held compressed by a gelatin coating which dissolves when the outer sheath is retracted and the gelatin comes into contact with fluids within the oesophagus. The system is introduced over an 0.035 inch stiff guidewire; proximal and distal radio-opaque markers aid accurate positioning.

Gianturco stent (Figure 5.2)

This stent has undergone several modifications since its introduction. The most recent design consists of a 0.5 mm wire of interlocking stainless steel in a zigzag configuration. This is coated with a polyethylene film and has central outer fixation barbs to reduce the risk of migration. The outer diameter in the central portion is 18 mm (inner diameter 16 mm) and both the proximal and distal ends are flared to 25 mm. The stent is available in lengths of 10, 12 and 14 cm and comes mounted in a 60 cm, 24 Fr introducer system. Radio-opaque markers delineate the proximal and distal ends of the stent to aid accurate positioning. The fully expanded stent is compressible in its radial axis but not longitudinally. The system is introduced over an 0.035 inch stiff guidewire.

Wallstent endoprosthesis (Figure 5.3)

The Wallstent is a self-expanding metallic mesh originally designed for use in the biliary tree. The basic design of the oesophageal Wallstent is the same as the device for biliary use but it has a larger calibre, its middle section is covered with

Figure 5.1   (a)

(a) The Ultraflex uncovered oesophageal stent. (b) Barium oesophagogram demonstrating free flow through an Ultraflex endoprosthesis positioned across a malignant lower oesophageal stricture. This endoprosthesis (arrows) is less radio-opaque than the other endoprostheses.

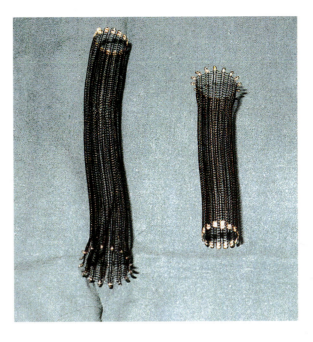

(b)

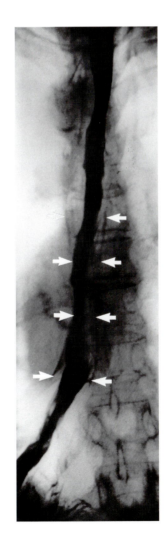

(a)

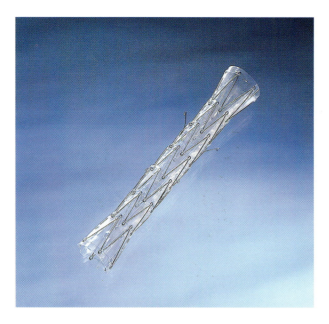

(b)

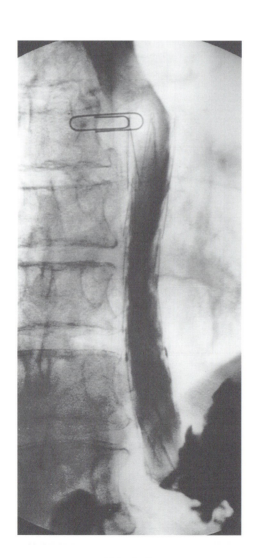

Figure 5.2
(a) The polyethylene covered Gianturco oesophageal stent. Note the central barbs to increase stability. (b) Barium oesophagogram demonstrating free flow through a Gianturco endoprosthesis positioned across a malignant lower oesophageal stricture.

Figure 5.3   (a)

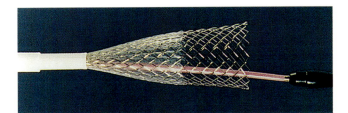

(a) The Wallstent oesophageal endoprosthesis. The central section is covered with polyurethane and the proximal and distal ends are uncovered to increase stabilty. The outer sheath has been withdrawn releasing 50% of the stent. Recovering and repositioning is possible as long as no more of the stent is released. (b) Barium oesophagogram demonstrating free flow through a covered Wallstent endoprosthesis positioned across a malignant oesophageal stricture. (Reproduced with permission from Watkinson AF et al. Esophageal carcinoma: initial results of palliative treatment with covered self-expanding endoprostheses. Radiology 1995; 195: 821–827)

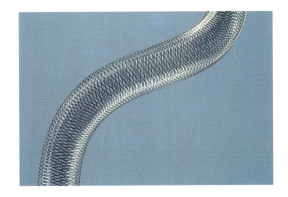

(b)

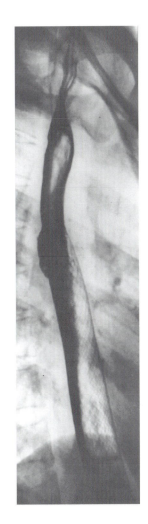

polyurethane and the details of the release mechanism are different. The oesophageal Wallstent endoprosthesis (Telestep device) comes in two sizes — 20 mm diameter, 110 mm long; and 25 mm diameter, 105 mm long — mounted on 18 Fr and 22 Fr delivery systems, respectively. The delivery system consists of three coaxially arranged shafts. The stent carrier is part of the inner shaft; this has a central lumen that accepts a 0.035 inch guidewire, assisting the coaxial introduction of the device across an oesophageal stricture. The stent is preloaded on the stent carrier, its position being indicated by radio-opaque markers adjacent to its proximal and distal ends. The outer sheath extends to the tip of the device and when withdrawn releases the distal 50% of the stent.

A distinct advantage of this stent over the previously described devices is that repositioning is possible if the position is unsatisfactory, provided that 50% or less of the stent has been released. The outer sheath can be readvanced over a partially released stent to allow repositioning as long as the middle sheath has not been withdrawn. The final step in the release of the stent is the withdrawal of the middle sheath, which completely frees the device. The stent shortens on release; the amount of shortening depends on the degree of expansion, the nominal length being reached on achieving the maximum calibre.

Stent insertion

The basic technique, apart from minor details particular to each stent design, is the same for all three devices. The Wallstent endoprosthesis is the only one that can be repositioned during deployment.

Equipment

1 Steerable catheter (biliary manipulation catheter; William Cook Europe, A/S Bjaeverskov, Denmark).
2 Guidewires:
   145 cm – 0.035 inch straight (Bentson; William Cook Europe, A/S Bjaeverskov, Denmark);
   150 cm – 0.035 inch angled guidewire (Terumo Europe N.V., 3001 Leuven, Belgium);
   260 cm – 0.035 inch stiff exchange wire (Amplatz; William Cook Europe, A/S Bjaeverskov, Denmark).
3 Balloon dilatation catheters, with 4-8 cm long balloons, up to 20 mm in diameter (Olbert 10 mm; Meadox Surgimed A/K DK 3660 Stenlose, Denmark and Microinvasive 15-20 mm Medi-tech Inc., Watertown, MA 02172, USA).
4 Choice of self-expanding metallic endoprostheses:
   (i)   uncovered 18 mm diameter 7, 10 or 15 cm long nitinol Strecker stent (Boston Scientific, Medi-tech Inc., Watertown, MA 02172, USA);
   (ii) polyethylene-covered 18 mm diameter 10, 12 or 14 cm long Gianturco-Rösch stent (William Cook Europe, A/S Bjaeverskov, Denmark);
   (iii) polyurethane-coverered 20 or 25 mm diameter, 105 or 110 mm long Wallstent (Schneider AG, Bulach, Switzerland).
5 Local anaesthetic spray and lubricating gel.

Pre-procedure assessment

A careful review of a recent non-ionic contrast examination (within 24–48 hours) is necessary to establish clearly the upper and lower limits of obstruction (Fig. 5.4a) and to demonstrate any associated fistulation or perforation. This may determine the choice of an uncovered or covered endoprosthesis.

Technique

A transoral route is used with the patient in the left lateral position. The oropharynx is anaesthetized with topical anaesthetic spray, and a mouthguard inserted. The patient is connected to a pulse oximeter and nasally administered oxygen, and intravenous analgesia and sedation are administered (fetanyl and midazolam). A 6.5 Fr catheter with a 45° angled tip (biliary manipulation catheter) is then inserted orally over a floppy-tipped guidewire (Bentson, William Cook Europe, A/S Bjaeverskov, Denmark) and advanced to the level of the lesion. Non-ionic contrast medium (to reduce the risk in the event of aspiration) is injected via the catheter to identify the upper level of the stricture (Fig. 5.4b) and the exact point of any perforation or fistula. A metallic marker is then positioned on the skin to mark the upper limit of the tumour, although frequently sufficient contrast material remains in the oesophagus to make this unnecessary. The catheter and guidewire combination is then manipulated through the stenosis or occlusion and advanced into the stomach. A hydrophilic guidewire (Terumo Europe N.V., 3001 Leuven, Belgium) makes it possible to traverse even the tightest of strictures.

In patients with complete occlusion, in whom contrast medium does not delineate the stricture, probing the site of the occlusion with a combination of an angled catheter and a straight hydrophilic wire will enable the guidewire and catheter to be advanced into the stomach. The catheter is then withdrawn slowly with non-ionic contrast medium infusing, to define the lower limit of the tumour. A second metallic marker is used to mark this point; again, in most instances, there is sufficient air and positive contrast medium in the stomach and lower oesophagus to make this unnecessary. A stiff exchange wire (Amplatz 260 cm 0.035 inch) is then advanced into the stomach and the catheter withdrawn. An Olbert catheter with a 10 mm balloon is used for gradual dilatation of the stricture using hand pressure. In the presence of perforation or fistula dilatation is limited to 10 mm in order to reduce the risk of extending the oesophageal tear. In the absence of fistula, larger balloons are used to dilate the stricture to a maximum diameter of 20 mm. A stent of appropriate size is selected to cover the entire length of the stricture. The choice of stent depends on personal preference, although the results of randomized trials may help to define when a covered or uncovered stent is indicated.[21] The stent, lubricated with xylocaine gel, is inserted over a stiff guidewire under fluoroscopic guidance. The radio-opaque markers of the introducer system and residual contrast medium enable accurate positioning of the device across the stricture (Fig. 5.4c). The release mechanisms of the Wallstent, Strecker and Gianturco–Rösch endoprostheses are all different. The Wallstent device has the advantage of allowing re-covering and repositioning until 50% of the stent has been released. The Strecker stent is coated in the central core of the delivery device with gelatin. It is neccessary to wait 5–10 minutes after removal of the outer sheath until the stent has completely detached from the delivery shaft and the gelatin dissolved. The expansile radial force of the Gianturco–Rösch and

(a)

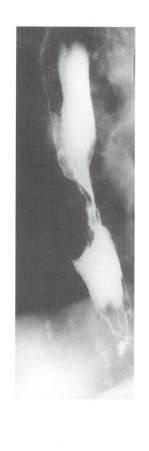

(b)

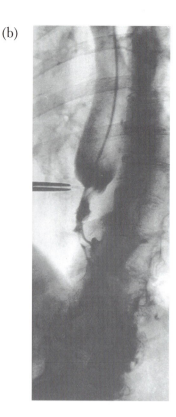

(c)

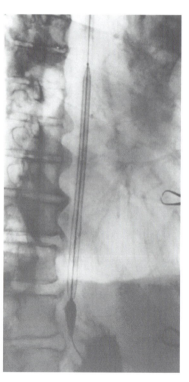

(d)

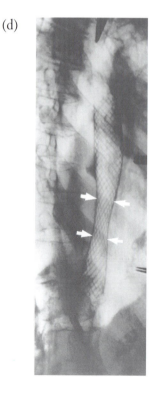

Figure 5.4
(a) A barium oesophagogram demonstrating a malignant stricture in the lower oesophagus. (b) An angled tip catheter has been introduced per-orally and advanced to the level of the stricture. Non-ionic contrast medium has been introduced to define the upper limit of the stricture. (c) An unreleased Wallstent has been introduced across the stricture, after balloon dilatation, over a stiff guidewire. Radio-opaque markers delineate the upper and lower limits of the contracted stent. (d) A covered self-expanding Wallstent has been introduced with 60% of the free stent above and 40% of the free stent below the stricture. Waisting (arrows) can be seen at the site of the stricture. ((d) reproduced with permission from Watkinson A F et al. Esophageal carcinoma: initial results of palliative treatment with covered self-expanding endoprostheses. Radiology *1995; 195: 821–827)*

Wallstent endoprostheses is significant, and postdilatation is rarely required. However, this is often necessary with the Strecker stent.

If the lesion is in the mid oesophagus, slightly more of the stent is left above the stricture than below (Fig. 5.4d) to counter the effects of peristalsis and reduce the risk of distal migration (Fig. 5.5). This is more important for covered than for uncovered stents. In patients with lesions very near to the gastro-oesophageal junction, the lower end of the stent must be left in the fundus of the stomach, just below the lower limit of the tumour, with most of the stent in the lower oesophagus (Fig. 5.6). In patients with long strictures, two overlapping stents may be required from the outset to achieve total coverage of the lesion.

Figure 5.5

(a) Lateral radiograph demonstrating non-ideal postioning of a covered oesophageal Wallstent. Waisting (arrows) is seen at the site of the stricture. Slightly more of the free stent is seen below the stricture than above. (b) A non-ionic contrast medium oesophagogram at the end of the procedure shows good flow through the endoprosthesis. (c) A barium swallow after 7 days shows there has been complete migration of the stent which is now lying in the stomach. (d) A CT scan 2 weeks after insertion of an oesophageal Gianturco endoprosthesis demonstrates that this has migrated into the second part of the duodenum. This required surgical removal. ((c) reproduced with permission from Watkinson A F et al. Esophageal carcinoma: initial results of palliative treatment with covered self-expanding endoprostheses. Radiology 1995; 195: 821–827)

(a)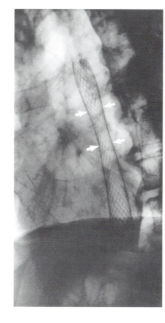

(b)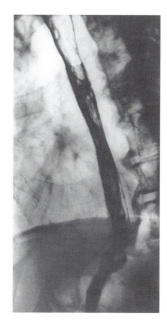

(c)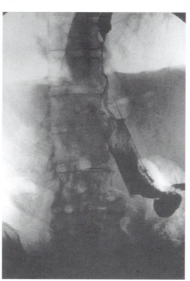

(d)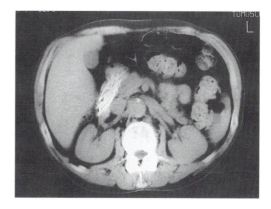

(a)

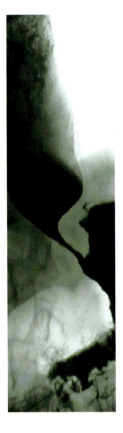

Figure 5.6
(a) A barium oesophagogram demonstrating a pseudo-achalasia appearance due to malignant stricture from an adenocarcinoma of the stomach extending into the oesophagus (biopsy proven).
(b) A Wallstent oesophageal endoprosthesis has been positioned with the lower end projecting into the stomach with the majority of the stent in the lower oesophagus. (Reproduced with permission from Watkinson A F et al. Esophageal carcinoma: initial results of palliative treatment with covered self-expanding endoprostheses. Radiology 1995; 195: 821–827)

(b)

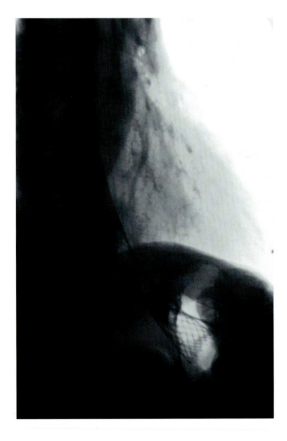

If a perforation or fistulation is present then a covered stent should be used (Fig. 5.7). The overall procedure time is approximately 30–45 minutes.

(a)

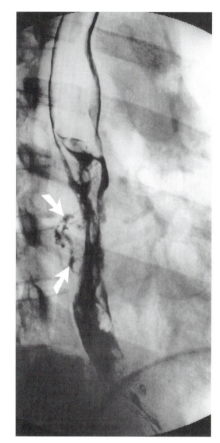

Figure 5.7
(a) A non-ionic contrast medium oesophagogram demonstrating a malignant oesophageal stricture associated with fistulation (arrows). (b) A contrast swallow after placement of a covered oesophageal Wallstent. There has been effective sealing at the site of leakage with free flow through the previously strictured segment.
(a) reproduced with permission from Watkinson A F et al. Esophageal carcinoma: initial results of palliative treatment with covered self-expanding endoprostheses. Radiology 1995; 195: 821–827)

(b)

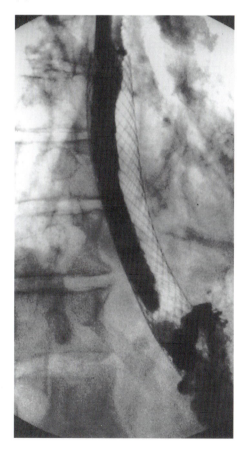

Aftercare

The patients are allowed to drink fluids 2–4 hours after the procedure once the local anaesthesia has worn off, and an oesophagogram is performed the following day. If there is free flow of contrast medium, with no extravasation, the patients are advised to commence a normal diet, although avoiding large lumps of solid food. Unless there are specific contraindications, all patients in whom the endoprostheses extend into the stomach should be commenced on omeprazole 20 mg daily (Prilosec; Astra Pharmaceuticals, Kings Langley, Herts, UK). This is to counter the effects of gastro-oesophageal reflux, which may be induced or worsened following stent insertion. Aggressive early treatment of any respiratory symptoms is needed if the stent is placed across the cardia, as these patients are prone to developing aspiration pneumonia.

If there is associated oesophageal perforation or a fistula, prior to stent placement, a strict regimen of nil by mouth, intravenous antibiotics (cefuroxime 750 mg tds, metronidazole 500 mg tds) and H2 receptor blockade is instituted. This regimen is maintained during and after stent insertion until the patient is clinically well (afebrile) and an oesophagogram has shown that the leak has stopped.

If early partial migration occurs, a second overlapping stent should be inserted to prevent further movement. If this is detected at the initial placement, a second stent should be inserted immediately. However, this may not be detected until 24 hours later, and a second stent should be inserted at the time of the check oesophagogram.

Recurrent dysphagia at a later stage, caused by tumour ingrowth or overgrowth, may occur depending on whether an uncovered or covered stent was inserted initially. The problem of tumour ingrowth is often solved by endoscopy where friable tumour is removed, following passage of the endoscope.[22] If this is unsuccessful, a second overlapping stent is inserted to re-establish oesophageal patency. A second overlapping stent is also inserted to solve the problem of tumour overgrowth.

Results and complications

Fluoroscopic stent placement is achieved in nearly 100% of patients,[14–24] with immediate improvement in dysphagia in 90–100%. Long-term palliation is achieved in over 80% of patients. Major complications are rare, with perforation secondary to stent insertion extremely uncommon.[14–24] Overall stent-related mortality is reported to be 0–6% and mostly relates to severe delayed upper gastrointestinal haemorrhage or aspiration pneumonia. Minor complications[14–24] include stent migration (0–30%), food impaction (6%), tumour overgrowth (5–10%), or ingrowth (5–50%) through the struts of uncovered stents. Gastro-oesophageal reflux is common, especially if the stent is left across the cardia, and varying degrees of central chest pain occur in 10–20% of patients; this is most common with the Gianturco–Rösch stent.

The disadvantage of tumour ingrowth in uncovered stents has to be balanced against the increased migration rate seen in covered stents which occurs in 10–25%.[18,21,23] New stent designs are currently being investigated to overcome these problems. The authors' own experience[18,20,21,22,24] suggests that covered stents are preferable for lesions in the upper, mid or lower oesophagus where the lower end of the stent is left above the cardia, and in patients in whom there is associated fistulation or perforation. Uncovered stents, however, are preferable for lesions at the cardia, as the migration rate is lower. The relative indications for the use of these newer techniques has become more clearly defined with the results of the authors' recently completed prospective, randomized trial.[21]

Conclusions

Results suggest that self-expandable metallic stents offer several advantages over conventional intubation and other palliative treatments. Insertion of stents is virtually always successful, with relatively few complications and excellent palliation of dysphagia. The low morbidity and mortality of insertion, compared with plastic endoprostheses, probably relates to the small calibre of the introducer system and the use of fluoroscopic guidance.

Stent insertion should be carried out under fluoroscopic guidance because:

1 It allows accurate localization of the upper and lower limits of the stricture.
2 Negotiation of difficult strictures is easier than with endoscopy. In the authors' experience of over 120 patients, many with complete dysphagia and failed endoscopy, the stricture was successfully traversed in every case.
3 Continuous visualization of the oesophagus, below the level of advancing catheters and guidewires, minimizes the risk of perforation.

Endoscopy is unnecessary in the vast majority of cases but, if a very high stent insertion is to be carried out, endoscopic visualization of cricopharyngeus may be helpful. Endoscopy alone is inappropriate for the insertion of oesophageal stents. It may be used in combination with good fluoroscopic facilities, but this would increase the cost of the procedure without any clinically significant benefits.

Problems are seen mainly in patients with lesions near the cardia, when the lower end has to project into the stomach. These patients have the highest incidence of stent migration, particularly if the stent is plastic covered. In this patient group the migration rate can be as high as 50%.[21] Although stent retrieval is possible using endoscopy and an overtube,[25] most stent manufacturers are currently working on new designs that are resistant to migration. In addition, patients in whom the stent projects into the stomach all suffer from gastro-oesophageal reflux, to a greater or lesser degree. This is helped symptomatically by H2 antagonists. Nevertheless, aspiration pneumonia is not an uncommon related complication, which can be fatal in this frail group of patients.

The later complication of recurrent dysphagia is best managed, at least initially, endoscopically. Food impaction is easily dealt with, and laser treatment is very effective for tumour ingrowth in uncovered stents. The tumour tissue is often friable and the passage of the endoscope will frequently brush the tissue away. If the problem is tumour overgrowth, either at the upper or lower end of the stent, then fluoroscopic placement of an overlapping stent will solve the problem in most instances.

There are two main disadvantages of metallic stents. The first is their cost, particularly if more than one stent is required to bridge the stricture or because of early migration. However, this must be balanced against improved palliation of symptoms and lower morbidity and mortality than is achieved with the plastic endoprostheses. In addition to benefiting the patient, this may be more economic in the long term, if the cost per patient is assessed, rather than the cost of an individual treatment episode. The second disadvantage is the high migration rate for covered stents inserted across the gastro-oesophageal junction[21] and the difficulty of removing these when necessary.

In the authors' institution a multidisciplinary team approach to each patient has been adopted for the palliation of inoperable oesophageal cancer. Both laser and metallic endoprostheses may be used in conjunction with other palliative treatments such as radiotherapy and chemotherapy.

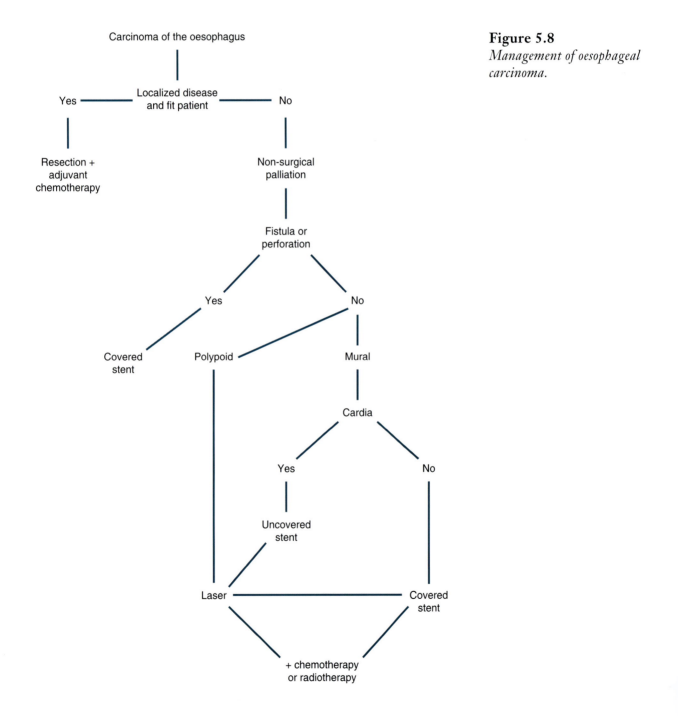

Figure 5.8
Management of oesophageal carcinoma.

The authors have just completed a triple randomized trial of Nd:YAG laser versus covered stent versus uncovered stent in the palliation of inoperable oesophageal malignancy. The early results of this study[21] suggest that in most instances self-expanding metallic stents give better palliation of the dysphagia associated with malignant obstruction. However, each case must be assessed individually to enable appropriate treatment to be given to achieve the best result.

Stents (both covered and uncovered) improve dysphagia and restore swallowing significantly better than endoscopic laser therapy.[21] Plastic-covered stents perform best in mural lesions in the middle third of the oesophagus, and are the device of choice when there is associated fistulation or perforation. Soft, uncovered stents are more suitable for high mural lesions, as they are less likely to cause unpleasant irritation, and also for lesions at the gastro-oesophageal junction, as they are less prone to migration. However, because of reflux and associated aspiration pneumonia it may be more appropriate to use laser as the initial management of gastro-oesophageal junctional tumours, with stents being reserved for laser failure at this site.

Laser is excellent at managing tumour ingrowth in stented patients. In addition, it is probably the treatment of choice for polypoid, rather than mural-based, oesophageal tumours. Figure 5.8 summarizes the authors' current views on the overall management of oesophageal carcinoma. It is a field of rapid technological advances, and self-expanding metallic stents have made a significant contribution to the management and palliation of dysphagia in a group of patients that has traditionally proved extremely difficult to treat.

References

1 Adam A, Watkinson AF, Dussek J. Boerhaave's syndrome: to treat or not to treat by insertion of a metallic stent. *J Vasc Intervent Radiol* 1995; **6**(5): 741–746.
2 Muller JM, Erasmi H, Stelzner M *et al*. Surgical therapy of oesophageal carcinoma. *Br J Surg* 1990; **77**: 845–857.
3 Earlam R, Cunha-Melo JR. Oesophageal squamous cell carcinoma: a critical review of surgery. *Br J Surg* 1980; **67**: 381.
4 Hishikawa Y, Kamikonya N, Tanakas S, Miura T. Radiotherapy of esophageal carcinoma: role of high dose rate intracavitary irradiation. *Radiother Oncol* 1987; **9**: 13.
5 Caspers RJ, Welvaart K, Verkes RJ. The effect of radiotherapy on dysphagia and survival in patients with oesophageal cancer. *Radiother Oncol* 1988; **12**: 15–23.
6 Atkinson M, Ferguson R, Parker GC. Tube introducer and modified Celestin tube for use in palliative intubation of esophago-gastric neoplasms at fibreoptic endoscopy. *Gut* 1978; **19**: 669.
7 Loizou LA, Grigg D, Atkinson M, Robertson C, Brown SG. A prospective comparison of laser therapy and intubation in endoscopic palliation for malignant dysphagia. *Gastroenterology* 1991; **100**: 1303–1310.
8 Fuegger R, Niederle B, Jantsch H, Schiessel R, Schulz F. Endoscopic tube implantation for the palliation of malignant esophageal stenosis. *Endoscopy* 1990; **22**: 101–104.
9 Mellow MH, Pinkas H. Endoscopic laser therapy for malignancies affecting the oesophagus and gastro-oesophageal junction: analysis of technical and functional efficacy. *Arch Intern Med* 1985; **145**: 1443–1446.
10 Brown SG. Endoscopic laser therapy for esophageal cancer. *Endoscopy* 1986; **18**: 26.
11 Mason RC, Bright N, McColl I. Palliation of malignant dysphagia with laser therapy: predictability of results. *Br J Surg* 1991; **78**: 1346–1347.
12 Houghton A, Mason RC, Allen A, McColl I. NdYAG laser treatment in the palliation of advanced oesophageal malignancy. *Br J Surg* 1989; **76**: 912–913.
13 Tyrrel M, Trotter G, Mason RC. The incidence and management of laser associated oesophageal perforation. *Gut* 1994; **35**: 59.
14 Knyrim K, Wagner HJ, Bethge N, Keymling M, Vakil N. A controlled trial of an expansile metal stent for palliation of esophageal obstruction due to inoperable cancer. *N Engl J Med* 1993; **329**: 1302–1307.
15 Song HY, Choi KC, Cho BH, Ahu DS, Kim KS. Esophago-gastric neoplasms: palliation with a modified Gianturco stent. *Radiology* 1991; **180**: 349–354.

16 Cwikiel W, Stridbeck H, Tranberg KG *et al*. Malignant esophageal strictures: treatment with a self-expanding nitinol stent. *Radiology* 1993; **187**: 661–665.

17 Song HY, Do YS, Han YM *et al*. Covered, expandable esophageal metallic stent tubes: experience in 119 patients. *Radiology* 1994; **193**: 689–695.

18 Watkinson AF, Ellul J, Entwisle K, Mason RM, Adam A. Esophageal carcinoma: initial results of palliative treatment with covered self-expanding endoprostheses. *Radiology* 1995; **195**: 821–827.

19 Do YS, Song HY, Lee BH *et al*. Esophagorespiratory fistula associated with esophageal cancer: treatment with a Gianturco stent tube. *Radiology* 1993; **187**: 673–677.

20 Watkinson AF, Ellul J, Farrugia M, Entwisle K, Mason RC, Adam A. Plastic-covered metallic endoprotheses in the management of oesophageal perforation in patients with oesophageal carcinoma. *Clin Radiol* 1995 **50**: 304–309.

21 Adam A, Saunders M, Tan B, Watkinson A, Ellul J, Mason R. Triple randomized comparison of laser therapy and two types of metallic stent in inoperable esophageal carcinoma: initial results. *Radiology* 1995; **197** (P): 347.

22 Ellul J, Watkinson A, Khan R, Adam A, Mason R. Self-expandable metal stents for the palliation of dysphagia due to inoperable oesophageal carcinoma. *Br J Surg* 1995; **82**: 1678–1681.

23 Saxon RR, Barton RE, Rösch J. Complications of esophageal stenting and balloon dilatation. *Semin Intervent Radiol* 1994; **11**(3): 276–282.

24 Watkinson A, Ellul J, Khan R, Mason RC, Adam A. Self-expandable metallic endoprostheses in malignant esophageal obstruction. SCVIR 1995; Fort Lauderdale Abstract Book **170**: 247.

25 Schaer J, Katon RM, Ivancev K, Uchida B, Rosch J, Binmoeller K. Treatment of malignant esophageal obstruction with silicone-coated metallic self-expanding stents. *Gastrointest Endosc* 1992; **38**: 7–11.

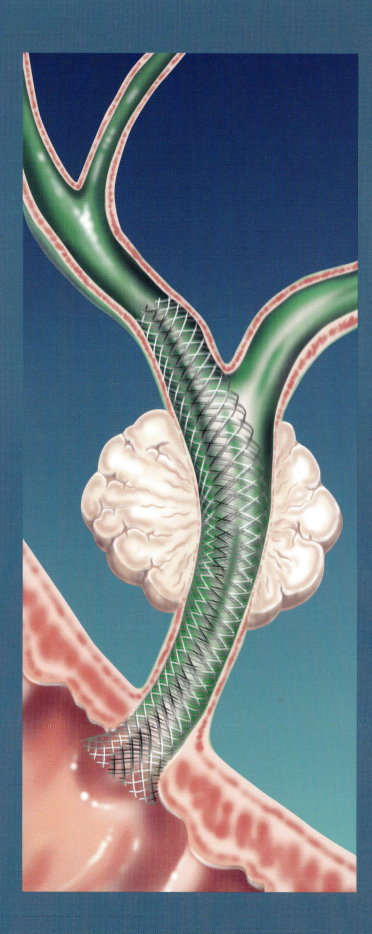

Chapter 6

Biliary metallic stents

B.L. Murphy, G.W. Boland and P.R. Mueller

Background

A stent (from Charles R. Stent, English dentist, died 1901) is defined as 'a slender rod- or thread-like device used to induce or maintain patency within a tubular structure'.[1] Since its first use in 1978, the search for the elusive perfect stent has been likened to the surfer's pursuit of the perfect wave.[2] The radiological placement of stents in the biliary tree evolved from the technique of external biliary drainage, first described by Molnar and Stockum in 1974,[3] which for the first time permitted access to the biliary tree without surgery. This landmark technique has since become the initial procedure for almost all radiologic biliary interventions, including stricture dilatation and stone retrieval in addition to stent placement.

The first description of percutaneous plastic stent placement in the biliary tree was by Burcharth in 1978,[4] with the first descriptions of endoscopic placement the following year.[5] Unfortunately, early results with plastic stents were poor, with early complications (mainly cholangitis) in up to 40% of patients and stent occlusion generally occurring approximately 3 months following placement.[6,7] Many factors were suggested as contributing to this early stent occlusion, including stent material and surface area, but the single most important factor was found to be the internal diameter of the stent. Larger-diameter stents allowed a higher flow of bile and reduced encrustation of bile salts.[8–11] This promise of increased long-term patency led to the development of larger-diameter plastic stents, which unfortunately resulted in an increase in the occurrence of complications and increased patient discomfort.[10]

The main advantages of plastic stents were their relatively low cost and the fact that they could be removed. Removal of the stents percutaneously can, however, be technically challenging and occasionally impossible, necessitating restenting with the original occluded stent remaining in place. It should be noted that plastic stents cannot be removed endoscopically unless they project beyond the ampulla into the duodenum. The concerns regarding stenting with metallic stents in benign disease do not apply to plastic stents since they are not incorporated into the wall of the bile duct. However, for the same reason, migration of plastic stents can occur at any time following their placement in 3–5% .[12–14]

The first reports of the results with metallic stents emanated from Europe and the USA in 1989.[15–17] These new stents, predominantly of a modified Gianturco (Cook, Inc., Bloomington, IN, USA) design, had small-calibre delivery systems that allowed for the placement of a stent much larger than the transhepatic track required for its delivery, in contrast to the large tracks previously required for plastic stents. Their lumina were enormous (30 Fr) compared with the plastic stent and their surface area, another important factor leading to bile salt encrustation, was minimal. The new metallic stents could not be removed, but were large enough to allow for reintervention through their lumen if required. Late migration was almost unheard of.

Although these stents were more expensive than their plastic predecessors, this high initial cost was balanced with the total cost of treatment, including potential replacement of the stent, as well as therapy and hospital stay for other complications. Two endoscopic studies have shown a *decreased* overall cost of treatment with metal stents when compared with plastic.[18,19]

It rapidly became apparent that metallic stent placement was more comfortable for the patient and more simple for the radiologist than plastic stent insertion. Successful initial drainage was possible in 95–100% of patients,[20-2] and migration occurred only during or immediately following the procedure.[21,23,24] Other direct comparisons between plastic and metallic stents are more difficult owing to the retrospective nature of most studies, and the combination of patients with benign and malignant disease, hilar and distal strictures and different types of stent.[25] Early results were variable.[20,21,26-8] However, it is now clear that metallic stent placement has a lower complication rate than plastic stent placement and that metallic stents remain patent longer than their plastic counterparts.

Early complications (Table 6.1), principally cholangitis, are seen in up to 10% of patients following metallic stent placement, compared with 10–30% for plastic stent placement.[21,26,29-31] The higher figures represent hilar tumours, which have increased early and late complication rates when compared with distal lesions. The principal late complication of stenting is recurrent jaundice due to stent

Complication	
Early (within 30 days of stent placement)	
Cholangitis	Commonest early complication. Severity ranges from mild fever to hypotensive collapse. May lead to hepatic abscess.
Haemobilia	Haemobilia requiring transfusion is the commonest major complication.
Bile peritonitis	Commonest with central approaches.
Pneumothorax	With right-sided transpleural approaches (above 10th rib). Rarely requires chest tube placement.
Migration	Rare. Occurs during or soon after placement. More likely with 'sleeve' technique.
Late	
Stent occlusion	Due to tumour overgrowth. Inevitable, but life of stent may be prolonged by careful placement. May present with severe sepsis.
Cholecystitis	Due to cystic duct obstruction. Consider percutaneous cholecystostomy.
Duodenal ulceration	With stent protruding into duodenum. May lead to perforation. Rare.

Table 6.1
Possible complications following stent placement.

occlusion. This is mainly caused by sludge in plastic stents, while tumour overgrowth due to spread of tumour along the ducts, rather than tumour ingrowth through the stent mesh, is the major factor leading to occlusion of metallic stents.[32-5] As one might expect, metallic stents remain patent longer than plastic stents because of this,[36,37] although precise patency figures are difficult to obtain because of the wide variety of study designs in the literature. It is clear from the available data, however, that recent results have improved substantially on early data and that long-term patency rates are higher in distal rather than hilar tumours.[20-2,26,28,30,31,33,39,40] Patency rates of 89% at 1 year have been obtained in common duct obstruction, with 1-year patency of only 46% for hilar obstruction in the same series.[39] In one relatively small series,[40] adequate palliation was achieved in 83% without further intervention. Interestingly, a large European series[28] demonstrated a significant difference in long-term patency between different types of metallic stent, the Wallstent™ (Schneider, Minneapolis, MN, USA) and nitinol Strecker (Boston Scientific Corporation, Watertown, MA, USA) stent outperforming the original Strecker and the Z-stent (25-week patency rates 67 and 78%, versus 30 and 20%, respectively).

Late cholangitis is less common with metal stents, occurring in 15% versus 36% with plastic stents,[38] and the 30-day mortality rate for metal stents is lower than both plastic stent placement and simple external drainage,[32] although this may be due to the poorer condition of those patients selected for external drainage alone.

Features of metal stents

There are several different types of metal stent available. The features of the various types are described below and summarized in Table 6.2.

Table 6.2
Technical features of five types of metallic stents

Stent	Type	Material	Length diameter (mm)	Delivery system diameter (Fr)	Other
Wallstent™	Self-expandable	Stainless steel mesh	20–94 10	7	Most popular metal stent
Gianturco–Rösch Z-stent	Balloon-expandable	Stainless steel zig-zag	15–90 6–12	10	Greatest inherent radial force
Palmaz	Balloon-expandable	Stainless steel lattice	10–39 4–12	7+	
Strecker (original)	Balloon-expandable	Tantalum mesh	40–80 4–12	5	Mainly vascular use
Nitinol Strecker (Accuflex)	Self-expandable	Nitinol mesh	40–60 10	10	Large delivery system

Wallstent

This is the most widely used metal stent both in the USA and in Europe. It is self-expandable (i.e. does not require balloon dilatation to achieve its maximal diameter) and flexible, and is manufactured from 18 stainless steel monofilaments. Its delivery system is, together with the Strecker, the smallest available at 7 Fr and lengths from 20 to 103 mm are available, having a maximal diameter of 8, 10 or 12 mm. It also has the advantage that two Wallstents may be inserted side by side in hilar obstruction. In contrast, balloon-expandable stents have no intrinsic radial expansile force and cannot be deployed in this fashion. Marked shortening of the order of 30% occurs as the stent reaches its final diameter (the length of the stent refers to its final length once expanded and not to its length on the delivery system prior to deployment), which may reduce the accuracy of final placement.

Prior to deployment the compressed Wallstent is mounted on a catheter inside a translucent covering sheath, which has a hydrophilic membrane. The stent is deployed by gradually retracting the covering sheath while the catheter is held still, allowing the stent to expand off the catheter. A comprehensive description of the technical and practical aspects of Wallstent insertion is given below.

At the time of writing, a new modification of the Wallstent delivery system has just been introduced in Europe under the tradename Placehit™. This system constrains the Wallstent with a simple 7 Fr sheath rather than the hydrophilic membrane system, and permits the stent to be reconstrained when up to three-quarters deployed, facilitating repositioning either proximally or distally. No preparation of the system is required, and a radio-opaque marker indicates the extent of maximal shortening. The stents will be available in 8 and 10 mm diameters and lengths of 5, 7 and 9 cm. This new design will replace the current hydrophilic membrane system.

Gianturco–Rösch Z-stent

This is a self-expandable, relatively rigid stent manufactured from a single stainless steel 0.018 inch wire with six zigzag bends. A suture encircles the ends of the stent to restrict expansion to a preselected diameter of 6, 8, 10 or 12 mm. Each stent measures 1.5 cm in length. If six stents are connected together, lengths of up to 9 cm can be achieved. The delivery system is a 10 Fr sheath with a pusher catheter. In contrast to the Wallstent, the delivery system is separate from the stent, which must be compressed and loaded by the operator into a sheath, via a peelaway sleeve. The stent is then pushed to the end of the sheath and deployed by withdrawing the delivery sheath.

Although the Gianturco–Rösch Z-stent has the greatest inherent radial force of the metal stents, the large areas of empty space associated with the design may predispose to tumour ingrowth, and occlusion has been reported in up to 67%.[28] A reduced long-term patency rate has been observed when compared with the Wallstent and nitinol Strecker stent (see above). A covered version may be more successful.[41]

Palmaz stent

The Palmaz (Johnson & Johnson, Warren, NJ, USA) is a balloon-expandable stent that is available either premounted on a balloon or separately. It consists of a stainless steel lattice of length 10–39 mm and diameter 4–12 mm (usually 8–10 mm in the biliary tree). The stent/balloon assembly will fit through a 7 Fr sheath, although larger sheaths may be required for stents of diameter 10 mm and greater.

The Palmaz stent is placed by inserting it, mounted on its dilating balloon, over an 0.035 inch guidewire through a sheath. The sheath is retracted when the stent is in position, and is deployed by inflating the balloon. Minimal shortening of the stent occurs, and the stent is entirely rigid, making placement around angles impossible. As it is not self-expandable, no further change in the stent will occur following its placement.

Strecker stent

This is a balloon-expandable stent made from a knitted mesh of a single tantalum wire. It is available in diameters from 4 to 12 mm and in lengths of 4–8 cm (the larger diameters are not available in 8 cm lengths). An introducing sheath of 7–9 Fr is required, depending on the final diameter of the stent. It is an extremely flexible stent but has no intrinsic radial force, and migration and collapse of the stent are therefore potential problems in the biliary tree.[28] The Strecker is most widely used as a vascular stent, where its flexibility is an obvious advantage.

Deployment of the Strecker stent is similar to that of other balloon-expandable devices. The stent is premounted on its balloon catheter (5 Fr) with a protective sleeve over it. An 0.035 inch guidewire is placed across the lesion and the system is advanced through a sheath and positioned appropriately. The protective sleeve is drawn back and the balloon is inflated to deploy the stent. Minimal shortening occurs, aiding correct positioning, and the soft looped ends of the stent should not damage ductal or bowel mucosa,[40] an occasional problem with the Wallstent.[27]

Accuflex Stent System (nitinol Strecker Stent)

Although this stent is of the same knitted single wire configuration as the Strecker, it is made from an elastic titanium-based alloy (nitinol) instead of tantalum. This renders it a self-expandable stent with a constant radial force rather than the balloon-expandable, zero radial force of the Strecker. The system consists of the compressed stent mounted on a delivery catheter, contained within a 10 Fr introducing sheath which covers the stent. This 10 Fr size is a disadvantage when compared with the 7 Fr of the Wallstent. It is currently available in 4 and 6 cm lengths, both of which are 10 mm in diameter when fully expanded. As noted previously, this stent may have the highest long-term patency rate among the metal stents.

Deployment is similar to the Wallstent. An 0.038 inch guidewire is placed across the obstruction and the stent system is positioned as desired. When the outer sheath is withdrawn, the stent begins to deploy from its distal end. Shortening of the order of 35% occurs after release,[40] but an interesting feature is the presence of stabilization wires at the distal end of the stent. These wires maintain the distal end of the stent in position during deployment, releasing it only when the stent is fully deployed and the mounting catheter withdrawn. Thus the stent shortens only from its proximal end, potentially allowing more accurate placement. Three radio-opaque markers are present on the delivery catheter to facilitate placement, indicating the proximal end of the compressed stent, the distal end of the stent (compressed and deployed) and the final position of the proximal end of the deployed stent. This is extremely helpful as the stent itself is only poorly radio-opaque.

Practical aspects of stent placement

The goal of stent placement is to achieve adequate internal biliary drainage for the longest possible time. The long-term patency of a stent in an individual patient is subject to many factors beyond the control of the radiologist, including the site, size and nature of the obstructing tumour, the presence of anatomical variants and the general health of the patient. However, many factors are within the control of the operator, an understanding of which leads to the formation of principles that may be applied to all patients in order to maximize the potential benefit to the individual patient. The application of these principles may help to prolong the life of the stent, to increase the success rate of the initial procedure thereby reducing the number of procedures (and therefore length of hospital stay) that the patient must undergo, and to reduce the risk of complication and early stent failure. This potentially leads to safer stent placement, which is more successful and less expensive.

Although stenting in benign disease has been described and is performed in a number of centres,[17,20,26,42,43] the known natural history of the metal stent appears to be occlusion after a finite period. Therefore, stenting in benign disease cannot be recommended without serious reservations. The following description refers to malignant biliary obstruction.

Pre-procedure investigation

The most important controllable factor in determining the short- and long-term success of biliary stent placement in malignant disease is the site at which the biliary tree is entered by the stent delivery catheter. This choice not only affects the segment(s), and therefore volume, of the liver that will be decompressed and drained, but also has a profound effect on the longevity of the stent. Overgrowth of tumour beyond the end of the stent is most often responsible for stent failure, while ingrowth of tumour leading to obstruction occurs rarely, if at all.[33–5,42] Therefore, the more peripherally a stent can be placed, the longer it is likely to remain patent before tumour overgrowth occurs. This 'overstenting' is the key to long-term success.[34] Another potential advantage of the peripheral entry site is a reduction in haemorrhagic complications.[44]

The duct(s) to be stented must also drain the maximum volume of *normal* liver. Liver segments that have become atrophic owing to long-term obstruction or are infiltrated with tumour or metastases are not suitable for drainage. Since these segments will frequently appear normal during fluoroscopy and cholangiography, it is imperative that the radiologist has access to the maximal relevant information prior to undertaking the procedure in order to make the most effective choice of access site.

Although it is possible to perform *external* biliary drainage in an emergency situation without extensive investigation, all patients undergoing internal biliary drainage with metallic biliary stent placement must be comprehensively evaluated radiologically before stent placement. CT is the modality of choice in this regard.

CT enables the level of obstruction to be delineated, allowing the radiologist to ascertain whether the obstruction is multisegmental, hilar, or of the common bile duct more centrally (Fig. 6.1 and Fig. 6.2). Patients presenting to the radiologist are likely to have multisegmental or superior common hepatic duct obstruction as the lower lesions are more frequently stented endoscopically. The

Figure 6.1
Example of pre-procedure imaging dictating best approach to a patient with periportal obstruction. (a) CT scan demonstrates dilated left ducts and large tumour in the porta (arrows). (b) Lateral spot during procedure. Stent was placed through an anterior left-sided drainage; good proximal position of the metallic stent is demonstrated. (c) Final film prior to withdrawal of safety catheter shows excellent final position of the metallic stent. The patient did well for 6 months prior to succumbing to his disease.

(a)

(b)

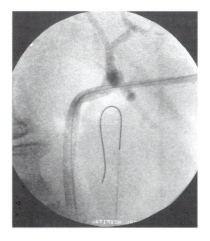

(c)

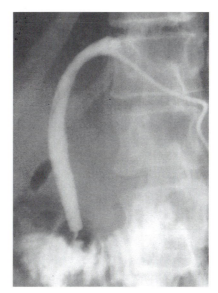

(a)

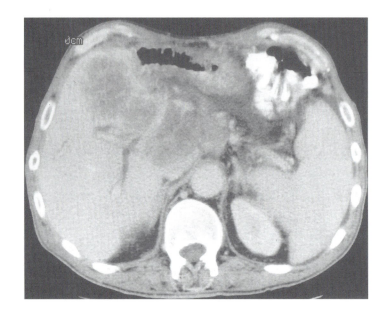

Figure 6.2
Metastatic carcinoma of the colon with invasion of liver segments II, III and IV.
(a) CT image demonstrating large metastases in segment IV. Note dilated duct in segment VI.
(b) Cholangiogram after drainage of segments V, VI, VII and VIII.

(b)

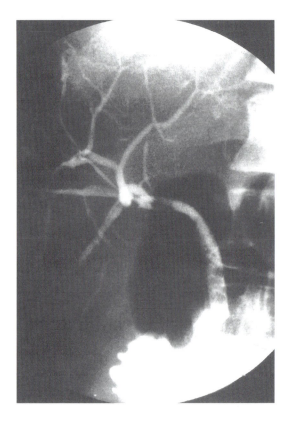

site of the lesion will influence the choice of a left- or right-sided approach, and will identify a suitable peripheral duct by which to attempt entry into the biliary tree. Atrophic liver segments and segments infiltrated with tumour will be demonstrated, the drainage of which may not significantly improve liver function. Anatomical variations, for example a high subcostal liver, that may cause difficulties with drainage may be identified and associated problems can then be anticipated. The position of abscess cavities can also be assessed and drainage of these can then be performed immediately under CT guidance. Unsuspected underlying liver disease, which may render the patient unsuitable for stenting, may be revealed.[44]

Although ultrasound can give most of this information, the availability of hard copy CT images, which include anatomical landmarks, during the procedure is invaluable. Pre-procedure ultrasound (US) scanning gives images that are helpful in some respects, but does not give an accurate guide as to the position of a particular duct in relation to overlying ribs, lung, pleura, etc. The major role of ultrasound is in guiding the site of initial puncture using real-time imaging to image the puncture needle directly in order to enter a chosen duct as peripherally as possible and, perhaps, to avoid major blood vessels.

Stent insertion

Ultrasound guidance

Puncture of the bile duct under direct real-time US guidance is particularly useful when a left-sided approach is employed, since there is usually no interference from overlying ribs, and when there is little or no duct dilatation present, as the operator is guided to a 'region of interest' in which to concentrate efforts to enter the duct, rather than the blind approach afforded by fluoroscopy alone. Direct US guidance has potential value in almost all cases, as it may reduce the number of transgressions of the liver parenchyma and also optimize the utility of the first puncture, frequently avoiding the need for a second needle placement.

Ultrasound guidance is also ideal for use with 'single stick' systems. Although these systems are very widely used and have the potential to allow a biliary procedure to be performed with only one bile duct puncture, they may encourage the operator to accept an entry site that is not as peripheral as could possibly be achieved. The use of US with the one stick type system will help to ensure that the initial puncture is as peripherally located as possible.

The second puncture

One should not hesitate to repuncture in cases where the initial puncture is not peripherally sited. When performing a second, more peripheral, puncture, it may be necessary to rotate the patient, if a C arm is not available, in order to determine the exact location of the ideal duct in the AP plane. An 18 G sheathed needle, which will accept an 0.038 inch guidewire directly, can then be advanced into a peripheral duct, eliminating the need for wire exchanges. The initial puncture needle is used to perform cholangiography and to distend the biliary tree if necessary and is left in place during the repuncture to provide alternate access if required.

Problems with the peripheral puncture

Difficulty may be encountered with the more peripheral entry sites when an acute angle is created, making advancement of a wire centrally or through a tight stricture difficult. A guidewire with a long distal 'floppy' portion can be used to form a loop directed inferiorly. It should then be possible to place a sheath to reduce the superior looping of the wire during manipulation, followed by a heavy-duty guidewire that should be placed well into the duodenum in order to maximize purchase. The heavy-duty wire in conjunction with the sheath will allow all but the tightest angles to be negotiated relatively easily.

It is important to state that the above considerations for choosing and entering the ideal access site do not apply in the emergency situation in patients with life-threatening cholangitis. In these patients the initial aim is simply to secure drainage and to allow infection to be brought under control. Stenting can then be performed on an elective basis, with a more peripheral puncture than that used to provide emergency drainage. With the more elective case, however, every effort should be made to access the biliary tree peripherally, since in this group of patients stenting can be performed at the initial procedure if the stricture has been successfully crossed without extensive manipulation. This single-procedure approach significantly reduces the length of hospital stay.[29]

Right- versus left-sided approach

The choice of a right-sided versus a left-sided approach is influenced by the position of the tumour. A low-lying lesion near to the ampulla can be stented from either approach; tumours located nearer to the confluence may be stented using bilateral stents in a T or Y configuration, while multisegmental obstruction is best approached from the left side (Fig. 6.3). A left-sided approach is recommended in multisegmental obstruction because a greater volume of viable liver tissue can be drained via this side and because there are fewer sidebranches near the confluence on the left side than on the right, which may mean that these will become obstructed with tumour later. This compares with the surgical approach to multisegmental biliary obstruction, the Bismuth procedure, in which the left duct system is surgically decompressed into the stomach.[29] A right-sided drainage and stenting can be performed at a subsequent procedure if cholangitis supervenes on this side.[45]

Stent positioning and deployment

Once the biliary tree has been accessed and the stricture has been crossed, a stent is placed with its peripheral end as close as possible to the biliary entry site,

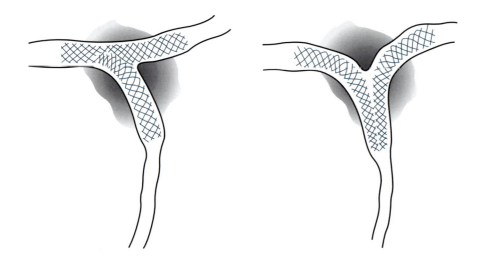

Figure 6.3
Schematic example demonstrating a double metallic stent placement depicting T- and Y-shaped metallic stent position.

taking extreme care that the peripheral end is not outside the duct in the liver (Fig. 6.4). A 'balanced' position is not as important as a peripheral position. A sheath should always be used to allow for safe retrieval of a faulty stent if problems arise during deployment and to allow safe balloon dilatation. The Wallstent delivery system has an outer diameter of 7 Fr and can be delivered through an 8 Fr sheath, although the new Wallstent design obviates the need for a sheath.

Figure 6.4
Clinical example of stent foreshortening. (a) Film from biliary drainage demonstrates initial position of percutaneous biliary drainage catheter. On this film it is difficult to delineate the exact area of entrance into the extrahepatic duct system. There is slight narrowing seen in the porta (arrows). (b) After insertion of the metallic stent, the proximal end of the stent is seen just below the narrowing from the tumour in the porta (arrows). (c) Pull-out injection demonstrating slight narrowing at the top of the stent (arrows) and what appears to be good flow of contrast from the extrahepatic duct system to the metallic stent. (d) Plain film demonstrating narrowing and pointing of the superior portion of the stent indicating that the proximal portion of the stent has foreshortened and may be within the tumour. The patient presented 3 months later with recurrent jaundice.

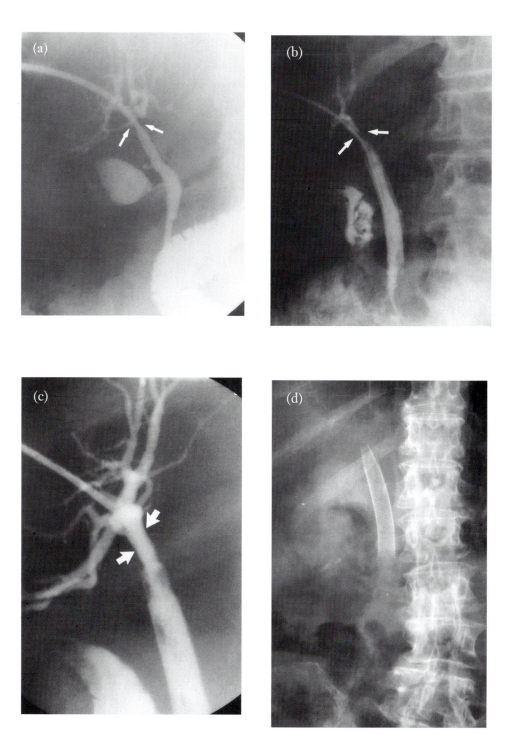

Careful consideration should be given to the effects of stent shortening when using self-expandable stents (Figs 6.5, 6.6, 6.7). The deployed Wallstent is some 30% shorter than when it is loaded on the delivery system, e.g. a 68 mm stent measures 100 mm prior to deployment. A stent reaches its final length about 10 days after deployment.[42] Allowance should be made for this, but a good rule of thumb is that if one is in doubt as to whether stent shortening will result in the peripheral end of the stent being in or near to the stricture, a repeat puncture should be performed with a second stent placement inside the first in a sleeve fashion. The radiological hallmark of the peripheral end lying in tumour is tapering of the stent. This sign also indicates tumour overgrowth rather than sludge as a cause for stent occlusion in the longer term.[29] Precise knowledge of the final position of the stent has been described as an advantage of balloon dilatation, and of non-self-expandable stents.[42]

(a)

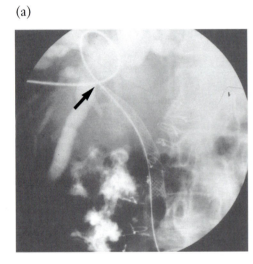

(b)

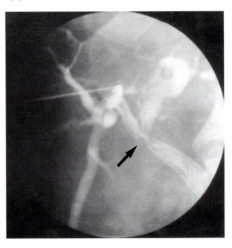

(c)

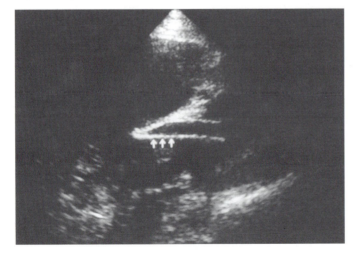

Figure 6.5
Example of poor initial purchase for placement of metallic stent. (a) The guidewire is seen entering the common duct close to the porta (arrow). The stent has already been placed. The proximal portion of the stent is barely within the dilated duct system. (b) Spot film after contrast has cleared shows the poor position of the proximal portion of the stent (arrow). (c) Ultrasound examination demonstrating the narrowed proximal stent (arrows). The patient did not drain well and eventually succumbed to sepsis and jaundice.

Figure 6.6
Schematic example of result of poor initial positioning of metallic stent. In this example the proximal portion of the stent has foreshortened into the area of the duct invaded by the tumour and become narrowed. The proximal ducts remain dilated.

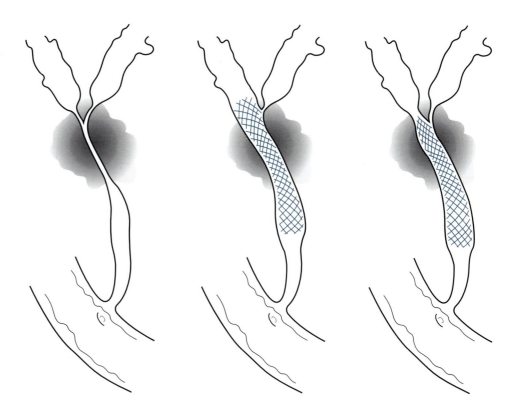

(a)   (b)

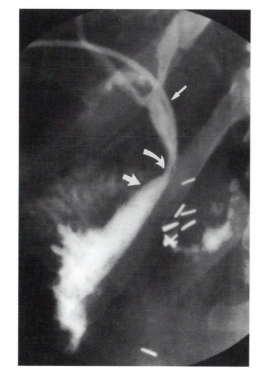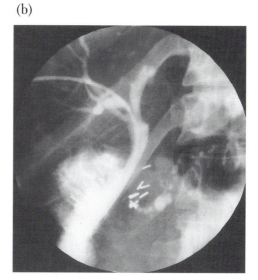

Figure 6.7
Example of stent that has slipped through a recurrent malignant stricture of a biliary enteric anastomosis so that the metallic stent no longer is draining. (a) The patient was redrained with a biliary catheter (arrows). Arrow demonstrates stent that has foreshortened and passed through the obstruction (arrows). (b) Image taken after placement of second metallic stent with proximal portion well within the intrahepatic duct system.

Balloon dilatation (of self-expandable stents)

The tumour can be balloon dilated prior to stenting, the stent can be balloon dilated after placement, or both can be performed (Fig. 6.8).[42] If a balloon is to be used, it is important to remember that full deflation of the balloon will not return it to its original diameter. The inelastic balloon will collapse into a transverse

(a)

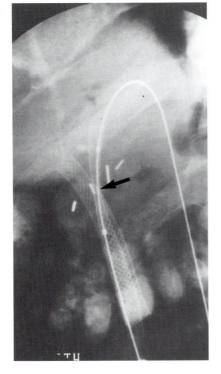

(b)

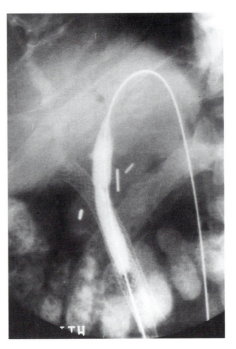

(c)

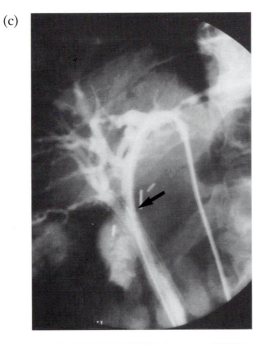

Figure 6.8
Example of use of percutaneous balloon dilatation to facilitate placement of metallic stent. (a) A right-sided metallic stent had been placed endoscopically. The left-sided stent was placed percutaneously; however, some narrowing of the metallic stent was seen in its mid-portion at the region of the porta (arrow). (b) A balloon was inserted over the guidewire and the metallic stent was subsequently dilated. (c) Final image immediately after dilatation of metallic stent shows further luminal widening which should allow better flow of bile (arrow).

Figure 6.9
Pre-procedure balloon dilatation. (a) Balloon dilatation prior to metallic stent placement demonstrates narrowing in an area of malignant stricture. (b) Film after placement of two metal stents shows good filling of the ducts and flow into the bowel.

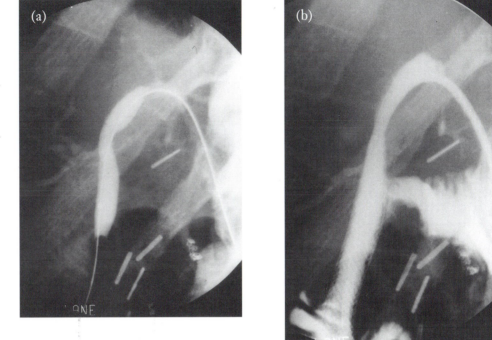

configuration of greater diameter than the uninflated balloon (Fig. 6.9). Therefore, although the balloon may be delivered through an 8 Fr sheath, it is frequently not possible to remove the balloon through this size of sheath. It may then be necessary to withdraw the balloon through the liver uncovered, leading to unnecessary trauma and increasing the likelihood of haemorrhage and infection. It is safest to use a 10 Fr sheath to deliver the balloon, although this theoretically increases the risk of haemorrhage and also restricts the options when considering a safety catheter.

If a stricture is very narrow, the placement of the balloon can push the newly sited stent centrally, leading to suboptimal positioning and unnecessary trauma to the biliary tree. In these patients, predilatation of the tumour will help to avoid this potential problem. The inflation of the balloon also prolongs the procedure and increases the risk of septicaemia and of haemorrhage, particularly with 10 mm diameter balloons;[45] an 8 mm balloon should therefore be used. In the authors' experience, balloon dilatation of the stent is not usually necessary in malignant obstruction as radial forces will expand the stent gradually over time.

After placement

A safety catheter should be placed after stenting. This has several important functions: it allows flushing of the stent to reduce clot formation; it allows for an alternative route of drainage immediately after stent placement; a 'trial of stent' function can be performed safely; a cholangiogram can be performed with ease; and direct access to the biliary tree is possible if further procedures are necessary. Additionally, the safety catheter will tamponade the track through the liver, provided that it is at least as large as the diameter of the track. The size of any safety catheter is therefore determined by the largest sheath or catheter used. Several choices are possible.

The simplest catheter to manage is a soft, straight, single-endhole catheter. The main advantage of this type of safety catheter is that it can be removed at the bedside without imaging or placement of a guidewire. It allows adequate external drainage, but does not drain the patient internally. It is easily dislodged and therefore not suitable for the uncooperative patient.

The other main choice for safety catheter is a multiple sidehole catheter with a loop in the duodenum acting as an anchor. This must be removed over a wire to avoid dislodgement of the stent, and fluoroscopic guidance is strongly advisable to ensure that the wire exits the catheter through the endhole rather than a sidehole, which could prove problematic if the catheter is then withdrawn with the pigtail still formed. When clamped, these tubes provide internal drainage and, perhaps, a false sense of security because clamping does not truly 'test' the stent.

Regardless of which is chosen, the safety catheter should be marked at the skin entry site with indelible ink so that migration can be readily assessed. It should be securely, but not tightly, affixed to the skin to avoid migration with respiration. A variety of suitable options are available, a good alternative being a stomadhesive ring, with the tube sutured to it via a 'flag' of adhesive tape. All safety catheters should be flushed regularly after placement. To assist with this, a three-way stopcock is placed between the safety catheter and the connecting tubing. Saline should be injected into the catheter *and* in the opposite direction, into the drainage bag. Aspiration should *not* be performed, as this may pull debris and clot into the catheter. The amount of saline used and the frequency of flushing the catheter is determined by the nature of the procedure. For example, a relatively atraumatic, bloodless procedure will require 10 ml N saline (5 ml to catheter, 5 ml to bag) every 4 hours reducing to every 8 hours, while a bloody procedure on a pus-filled biliary tree may require 20 ml/h initially. Regular assessment of the patient is vital to assess the need for any change in this regimen in addition to monitoring of the patient's condition.

The importance of rounds

Regular ward rounds by the interventional team are of paramount importance in the success of any catheter-based procedure.[46] The frequency of visiting a particular patient depends upon the procedure, but every biliary drainage patient should be seen 1, 4 and 12 h post-procedure and then at least once daily until the safety catheter is removed. This should be increased appropriately in difficult cases.

On rounds the patient is assessed clinically and changes in vital signs noted. The patient is asked if he/she has any complaints, specifically pain. The quantity and character of safety catheter drainage is noted. The position of the safety catheter is checked. Post-procedure orders can then be altered appropriately and a check can be made with the nursing staff to ensure that no difficulties exist with the carrying out of current orders. A typical order set will include the monitoring of vital signs every 15 min initially, gradually reducing to 4-hourly over the first 24 h, careful instructions on the flushing of the safety catheter, instructions to monitor the output of the safety catheter and to record its volume, and instructions to call the IR team with questions or problems. This can be added to appropriately, e.g. measurement of haematocrit in bloody procedures.

In addition to providing early warning of potential problems, regular rounds enable a closer doctor–patient relationship to develop, and allow for a closer relationship with clinical colleagues with whom the patient may be discussed at the bedside. It is also surprising how many referrals for new patients are obtained during these rounds!

Following stent placement, if the patient is stable and no unforeseen problems have arisen, the safety catheter can be clamped the next day. Instructions are given to the nursing staff and to the patient to note pain, leakage around the safety catheter at the skin site, signs of fever or other unexplained symptoms that may indicate obstruction. If these occur, the catheter should be unclamped and a cholangiogram performed when the patient's condition allows. If the patient is asymptomatic, the safety catheter can be removed after a 24 h period of observation following clamping of the catheter. Note that some do not recommend clamping of the catheter to test the stent, opting instead for a cholangiogram and immediate removal of the catheter.[45]

Multiple stent placement

Two or more stents may be placed either simultaneously during the initial stenting procedure, soon after the initial procedure to improve an unsatisfactory result, or in the longer term to obtain drainage when advancing disease has led to further obstruction.

Simultaneous stenting is most commonly performed when there is obstruction to the common hepatic duct at or near the confluence of the right and left hepatic ducts (Fig. 6.10). It is not possible to deploy non-expandable stents simultaneously. All of the above techniques may be employed in establishing drainage by the most peripheral puncture site possible. It is easier to perform the

Figure 6.10

Example of placement of two left-sided stents in patient with periportal obstruction. (a) Cholangiogram demonstrates left duct obstruction; right-sided stent was placed endoscopically. (b) Two left-sided stents were placed to bridge the obstruction.

(a)

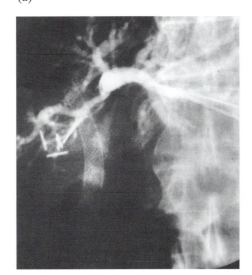

(b)

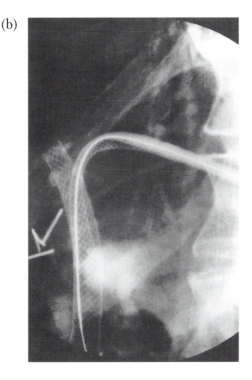

left-sided drainage before the right as repositioning of the patient is less likely to be impeded by a left-sided catheter. A catheter with a locking pigtail should be placed to reduce the chance of displacement.

Once bilateral biliary drainage catheters are in place, they are exchanged for heavy-duty guidewires, sheaths, and stent delivery catheters. The stents are positioned appropriately, and deployed simultaneously by two operators in a Y configuration (Fig. 6.3). Deployment is stopped every 1 cm approximately or, if one stent is becoming displaced, to allow the position of each stent to be optimized. Bilateral safety catheters can then be placed.

An alternative that can be used to perform bilateral drainage from a single approach is to place two stents in a T configuration. The horizontal portion of the T is a stent placed from the right system to the left main hepatic duct. A second stent is then placed through the mesh of the first from the right side into the common bile duct below the obstruction, forming the vertical portion of the T. This is extremely useful when left-sided access is difficult.[22]

In cases of an unsatisfactory initial result, it is usually a simple procedure to place a second stent inside the first in a 'sleeve' fashion, the second stent lying with its peripheral end more peripheral than the first (Fig. 6.11). If the original entry site, and therefore the safety catheter, is sufficiently peripherally sited, it is a simple matter to exchange the safety catheter for a sheath/stent delivery catheter system over a heavy-duty guidewire and to deploy the stent in the usual fashion. However, a second more peripheral puncture site should be chosen without hesitation if any doubt exists as to the suitability of the position of the first site. The safety catheter is then used to perform a cholangiogram to enable puncture of the same duct in which the stent lies. Although the bile ducts may not be distended at this stage if drainage has been satisfactory, a degree of distension can be achieved by simultaneous injection of the safety catheter during probing

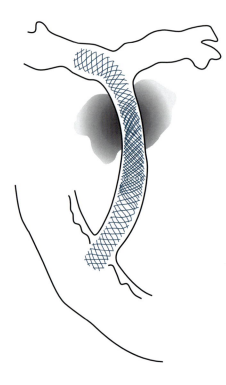

Figure 6.11
Schematic depiction of 'sleeve' stent (one stent placed within a second stent) to ensure better drainage.

with an 18G sheathed needle of a single-stick type system. The increased risk of infection with overzealous contrast injection should be considered. Biplane or C-arm fluoroscopy is not necessary as the patient can easily be repositioned in order to optimize the plane of entry into the duct system. Once the duct has been entered, the passage of the guidewire can be facilitated by further careful distension of the ducts by contrast injection.

When attempting to pass the guidewire through the stent, it is important to ensure that the wire has not inadvertently passed outside the stent, between it and the wall of the bile duct. A tight radius (3 mm) 'J' guidewire is ideal as it will rotate 360° without distortion if it is inside the stent, and is less likely to find a path outside the stent than a curved hydrophilic wire, for example. The wire may enter the top of the stent but exit through the mesh of the stent inferiorly. Although this position is salvageable if the stent is inadvertently deployed, this situation can again be avoided by careful use of a tight radius J wire. Once the initial stent has been successfully traversed, the original safety catheter is removed and the stent is deployed in the usual fashion. Additional caution is required as the original stent will provide little friction and it is easy for the second stent to slip through the first in a 'telescope' fashion, becoming displaced inferiorly.[22]

The blocked stent

In most patients who survive long term, stent blockage is a problem. When this is due to dehydration and sludge formation, hospital admission with rehydration and antibiotics may be sufficient. However, redrainage and 'dredging' of the stent with a balloon will frequently be necessary. If blockage of the stent is due to advancing disease, further drainage and stenting may be required (Fig. 6.12). It needs to be emphasized, however, that a rational approach to quality-of-life issues must be employed and further potentially painful, potentially unsuccessful procedures may not be in the best interests of the patient. External biliary drainage may be preferable in many cases.[34]

Once a decision has been made to proceed with drainage, initial external drainage, with or without crossing the obstruction, suffices initially. Once the patient is able to tolerate formal stenting, there are two options — the sleeve technique and the technique of stenting through the mesh of the existing stent.

It is frequently not possible to enter the same duct in which the original stent lies. If an emergency drainage has been performed, it is necessary to use the same duct to place the new stent, as this duct must be considered infected. In elective cases, an assessment is made as to the approachable duct that drains the largest segment(s) of liver, as for the original drainage described above. It is then frequently possible to provide drainage by stenting through the mesh of the original stent.

Using standard technique, a guidewire is manipulated through the side mesh of the stent. An 0.018 inch platinum-tipped or an 0.038 inch hydrophilic wire are usually suitable. A curved catheter is then used to direct the wire 'downstream'. A tissue dilator can be used to disrupt the mesh, followed by a 10 mm angioplasty balloon. Once a suitable hole has been dilated in the original stent, the second stent is deployed in the usual fashion.

In conclusion, careful attention to several key principles will help to increase long-term patency of metallic biliary endoprostheses. The stent should be placed

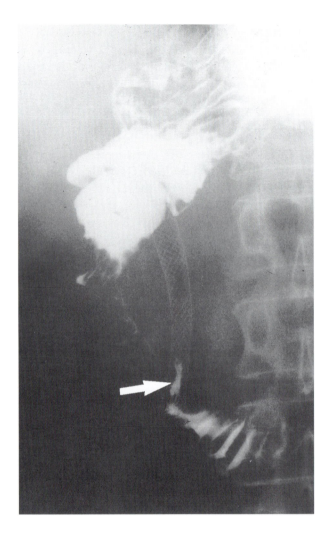

Figure 6.12
Example of tumour overgrowth in the duodenum, causing secondary obstruction of the stent. Film from an upper GI demonstrates irregular second portion of the duodenum consistent with pancreatic tumour overgrowth. This stent was dilated and patent (arrow).

as peripherally as possible in a duct that will drain the largest possible volume of normal liver. Pre-procedure investigation is an invaluable aid in this regard, and direct ultrasound guidance may be helpful. A second more peripheral puncture should be performed without hesitation if the initial puncture is unsatisfactory. Balloon dilatation should be performed judiciously, and consideration given to predilatation. Once the stent has been placed, the importance of regular ward rounds cannot be overestimated.

The future

Thus far, many attempts have been made to achieve prolonged stent patency, none of which have gained a wide acceptance. These have included covering the Gianturco stent with material to fill the mesh,[41] using a polymer coating to reduce bacterial adherence,[47] and the administration of choloretic agents to reduce sludge formation.[48] Innovative approaches to stent placement have included placement via a T-tube track,[49] or by a cholecystostomy,[50] and even perorally without endoscopy.[51] The metallic stent has been proposed as a possible site for the delivery of therapeutic ultrasound.[52] However, none of these approaches are likely to have the same impact as the introduction of the metallic stent itself.

In the longer term, refinements of the delivery systems and of stent materials will be developed and perhaps the 'perfect wave' will eventually sweep the 'surfers' on to the beach. It should be remembered, however, that obstructing biliary tumours continue to have a truly dismal prognosis and real advances in the treatment of these tumours are likely to lie outside the field of interventional radiology.

References

1   Taylor EJ (ed.) *Dorland's Illustrated Medical Dictionary*, 28th edition Philadelphia: WB Saunders Co., 1994.

2   Mueller PR. Metallic endoprostheses: boon or bust? *Radiology* 1991; **179**: 603–605.

3   Molnar W, Stockum AE. Relief of obstructive jaundice through percutaneous transhepatic catheter – a new therapeutic method. *AJR* 1974; **122**: 356–367.

4   Burcharth F. A new endoprosthesis for nonoperative intubation of the biliary tract in malignant obstructive jaundice. *Surg Gynecol Obstet* 1978; **146**: 76–78.

5   Soehendra N, Reynders-Frederix V. Palliative bile duct drainage. A new endoscopic method of introducing a transpapillary drain. *Endoscopy* 1980; **12**: 8–11.

6   Deviere J, Baize M, Buset M *et al*. Les complications du drainage biliaire interne endoscopique. *Acta Endoscopica* 1986; **16**: 19–29.

7   Gilbert DA, DiMarino AJ, Jensen DM *et al*. Status evaluation: biliary stents. *Gastrointest Endosc* 1992; **38**: 750–752.

8   Groen AK, Out T, Huibregste K, Delzenne B, Hoek FJ, Tytgat GNJ. Characterization of the content of occluded biliary endoprostheses. *Endoscopy* 1987; **19**: 57–59.

9   Leung JWC, Ling TKW, Kung JLS, Vallance-Owen J. The role of bacteria in the blockage of biliary stents. *Gastrointest Endosc* 1988; **34**: 19–22.

10 McLean GK, Burke DR. The role of endoprostheses in the management of malignant biliary obstruction. *Radiology* 1989; **170**: 961–967.

11 Dowidar N, Kolmos HJ, Lyon H, Matzen P. Clogging of biliary endoprostheses. A morphologic and bacteriologic study. *Scand J Gastroenterol* 1991; **26**: 1137–1144.

12 Mueller PR, Ferrucci JT, Teplick SK *et al*. Biliary stent endoprosthesis: analysis of complications in 113 patients. *Radiology* 1985; **156**: 637–639.

13 Lammer J, Neumayer K. Biliary drainage endoprostheses: experience with 201 placements. *Radiology* 1986; **159**: 625–629.

14 Dick BW, Gordon RL, LaBerge JM, Doherty M, Ring EJ. Percutaneous transhepatic placement of biliary endoprostheses: results in 100 consecutive patients. *J Vasc Intervent Radiol* 1990; **1**: 97–100.

15 Dick R, Gillams A, Dooley JS, Hobbs KE. Stainless steel mesh stents for biliary strictures. *J Intervent Radiol* 1989; **4**: 95–98.

16 Coons HG. Self-expanding stainless steel biliary stents. *Radiology* 1989; **170**: 979–983.

17 Irving JD, Adam A, Dick R, Dondelinger RF, Lunderquist A, Roche A. Gianturco expandable metallic stents: results of a European clinical trial. *Radiology* 1989; **172**: 321–326.

18 Knyrim K, Wagner HJ, Pausch J, Vakil N. A prospective, randomized, controlled trial of metal stents for malignant obstruction of the common bile duct. *Endoscopy* 1993; **25**: 207–212.

19 Wagner HJ, Knyrim K, Vakil N, Klose KJ. Plastic endoprostheses versus metal stents in the palliative treatment of malignant hilar biliary obstruction: a prospective randomized trial. *Endoscopy* 1993; **25**: 213–218.

20 Lammer J, Klein GE, Kleinert R, Hausegger K, Einspieler R. Obstructive jaundice: use of expandable metal endoprosthesis for biliary drainage. *Radiology* 1990; **177**: 789–792.

21 Adam A, Chetty N, Roddie M, Yeung E, Benjamin IS. Self expandable stainless steel endoprostheses for treatment of malignant bile duct obstruction. *AJR* 1991; **156**: 321–325.

22 Lee MJ, Dawson SL, Mueller PR *et al*. Percutaneous management of hilar biliary malignancies with metallic endoprostheses: results, technical problems and causes of failure. *Radiographics* 1993; **13**: 1249–1263.

23 Asch MR, Jaffer NM, Baron DL. Migration of a biliary Wallstent into the duodenum. *J Vasc Intervent Radiol* 1993; **4**: 381–383.

24 Abramson AF, Javit DJ, Mitty HA, Train JS, Dan SJ. Wallstent migration following deployment in right and left bile ducts. *J Vasc Intervent Radiol* 1992; **3**: 463–465.

25 Lameris JS, Stoker J. Metal stents for malignant biliary obstruction. *Dig Dis* 1994; **12**: 161–169.

26 Gillams A, Dick R, Dooley JS, Wallsten H, El-Din A. Self expandable stainless steel braided endoprosthesis for biliary strictures. *Radiology* 1990; **174**: 137–140.

27 Lameris JS, Stoker J, Nijs HGT *et al*. Malignant biliary obstruction: percutaneous use of self-expandable stents. *Radiology* 1991; **179**: 703–707.

28 Rossi P, Bezzi M, Rossi M *et al*. Metallic stents in malignant biliary obstruction: results of a multicenter European study of 240 patients. *J Vasc Intervent Radiol* 1994; **5**: 279–285.

29 Lee MJ, Dawson SL, Mueller PR, Krebs TL, Saini S, Hahn PF. Palliation of malignant bile duct obstruction with metallic endoprostheses: technique, results and complications. *J Vasc Intervent Radiol* 1992; **3**: 665–671.

30 Stoker J, Lameris JS, van Blankenstein M. Percutaneous metallic self-expandable endoprostheses in malignant hilar biliary obstruction. *Gastrointest Endosc* 1993; **39**: 43–49.

31 Stoker J, Lameris JS, Jeekel J. Percutaneously placed Wallstent endoprosthesis in patients with malignant distal biliary obstruction. *Br J Surg* 1993; **80**: 1185–1187.

32 Coons H. Metallic stents for the treatment of biliary obstruction: a report of 100 cases. *Cardiovasc Intervent Radiol* 1992; **15**: 367–374.

33 Stoker J, Lameris JS. Complications of percutaneously inserted biliary Wallstents. *J Vasc Intervent Radiol* 1993; **4**: 767–772.

34 Lee MJ, Dawson SL, Mueller PR *et al*. Failed metallic biliary stents: causes and management of delayed complications. *Clin Radiol* 1994; **49**: 857–862.

35 Boguth L, Tatalovic S, Antonucci F, Heer M, Sulser H, Zollikofer CL. Malignant biliary obstruction: clinical and histopathologic correlation after treatment with self-expanding metal prostheses. *Radiology* 1994; **192**: 669–674.

36 Davids PH, Groen AK, Rauws EAJ, Tytgat GN, Huibregste K. Randomised trial of self-expanding metal stents versus polyethylene stents for distal malignant biliary obstruction. *Lancet* 1992; **340**: 1488–1492.

37 Wagner HJ, Knyrim K, Vakil N, Klose KJ. Plastic endoprostheses versus metal stents in palliative treatment of malignant hilar biliary obstruction. A prospective and randomized trial. *Endoscopy* 1993; **25**: 213–218.

38 Knyrim K, Wagner HJ, Pausch J, Vakil N. A prospective, randomized, controlled trial of metal stents for malignant obstruction of the common bile duct. *Endoscopy* 1993; **25**: 213–218.

39 Becker CD, Glattli A, Maibach R, Baer HU. Percutaneous palliation of malignant obstructive jaundice with the Wallstent endoprosthesis: follow-up and reintervention in patients with hilar and non-hilar obstruction. *J Vasc Intervent Radiol* 1993; **4**: 597–604.

40 Bezzi M, Orsi F, Salvatori FM, Maccioni F, Rossi P. Self-expandable nitinol stent for the management of biliary obstruction: long term clinical results. *J Vasc Intervent Radiol* 1994; **5**: 287–293.

41 Yasumori K, Mahmoudi N, Wright KC, Wallace S, Gianturco C. Placement of covered self-expanding metallic stents in the common bile duct: a feasability study. *J Vasc Intervent Radiol* 1993; **4**: 773–778.

42 Salmonowitz EK, Antonucci F, Heer M, Stuckmann G, Egloff B, Zollikofer CL. Biliary obstruction: treatment with self-expanding metal prostheses. *J Vasc Intervent Radiol* 1992; **3**: 365–370.

43 Vorwerk D, Kissinger G, Handt S, Gunther RW. Long term patency of Wallstent endoprostheses in benign biliary obstructions: experimental results. *J Vasc Intervent Radiol* 1993; **4**: 625–634.

44 Venbrux AC, Osterman FA. Percutaneous transhepatic cholangiography and biliary drainage: step by step. In: LaBerge JM, Venbrux AC (eds) *Biliary Interventions*. SCVIR Syllabus Series, 1995.

45 Gordon RL, Ring EJ, LaBerge JM, Doherty MM. Malignant biliary obstruction: treatment with expandable metallic stents — follow-up of 50 consecutive patients. *Radiology* 1992; **182**: 697–701.

46 Goldberg MA, Mueller PR, Saini S *et al*. Importance of daily rounds by the radiologist after interventional procedures of the abdomen and chest. *Radiology* 1991; **180**: 767–770.

47 Hoffman BJ, Cunningham JT, Marsh WH, O'Brien JJ, Watson J. An in vitro comparison of biofilm formation on various biliary stent materials. *Gastrointest Endosc* 1994; **40**: 581–583.

48 Barrioz T, Ingrand P, Besson I, de Ledinghen V, Silvain C, Beauchant M. Randomised trial of prevention of biliary stent occlusion by ursodeoxycholic acid plus norfloxacin. *Lancet* 1994; **344**: 581–582.

49 Kim JK, Kim HJ, Kim HK *et al*. Percutaneous placement of biliary stent through T-tube tract. *Abdom Imaging* 1994; **19**: 512–514.

50 Dawson SL, Girard MJ, Saini S, Mueller PR. Placement of a metallic biliary endoprosthesis via cholecystostomy. *AJR* 1991; **157**: 491–493.

51 Bley WR, Ahmad I. Peroral radiographic placement of biliary stents. *J Vasc Intervent Radiol* 1992; **3**: 375–377.

52 Goldberg SN, Ryan TP, Gazelle GS, Lawes KR, Dawson SL, Mueller PR. RF tissue ablation: transluminal application via metallic stents (abstract). *Radiology* 1995; **197** (P): 382.

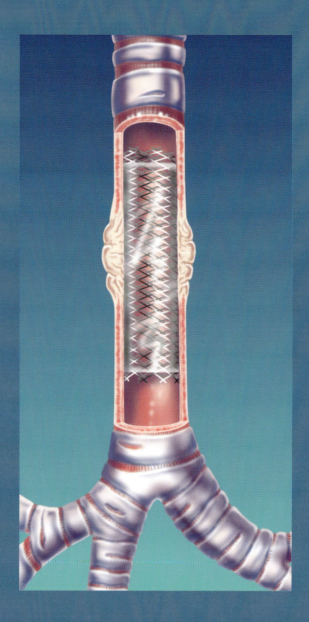

Chapter 7

Endoprostheses in the tracheobronchial system

D. Liermann, H.D. Becker and M. Rust

Introduction

Tracheobronchial stenoses are a relatively common condition. In addition to agenesis and atresia of the trachea and anomalies of isolated segmental bronchi, there are several other causes of bronchial stenoses. Double aorta, which can compress the trachea, deserves special mention, as it causes progressive stenosis with tracheomalacia.[1–8] Such changes, which can already be present during infancy, are usually recognized through secondary phenomena such as stridor or recurrent pneumonia caused by impaired ventilation. This also applies to deformed constricted segmental bronchi, which must be treated as soon as possible.[2,10–15]

In the event of acute occlusion, there are only a few minutes available for removal of the obstruction, insertion of a tracheal tube, or performance of a tracheotomy. The management of tracheobronchial stenoses is less dramatic but equally vital. It is important to distinguish between extrinsic and intrinsic bronchial stenoses and occlusions. Cystic fibrosis, a systemic disease of the exocrine glands, results in a thickening of the mucus that leads to blockage of peripheral and segmental bronchi,[16] particularly in older patients and those inadequately treated. Cystic fibrosis cannot be treated by recanalization or dilatation. Similarly in other conditions characterized by increased mucus production and an inability to expectorate repeatedly, it is usually possible to remove the blockage adequately by medication or aspiration.[16] In the case of benign compressive conditions accompanied by respiratory insufficiency, such as retrosternal goitre, tracheomalacia, localized strictures or constriction resulting from iatrogenic injury, the long life expectancy favours the selection of surgical methods.[17–24,26]

The situation is completely different in the case of malignant endoluminal tumours, or tumours infiltrating and penetrating the lumen from the outside.[27–31] Here, palliative therapy is required to maintain adequate respiratory function of the longest possible period. In these cases, the emphasis is frequently placed on a combined application of alternative methods such as laser, percutaneous balloon dilatation, endoluminal splinting, endoluminal afterloading therapy, percutaneous irradiation, and chemotherapy.[18,20,24,32,34,35] A further addition to the range of alternative methods of treatment consists in the use of self-expanding and balloon-expandable stents for the treatment of tracheobronchial stenoses. Compared with surgical treatment of stenoses in the trachea, stent application is a simple method, resulting in immediate improvement in the quality of life. This is the main goal of treatment, particularly in the case of malignant stenoses with limited life expectancy.

Metallic stents

The thickness of the wall compared with the diameter is negligible in metallic stents. There are basically two types of metallic stents — balloon-expandable and self-expanding systems. The balloon-expandable systems, mainly the Palmaz® stent (Johnson & Johnson Interventional Systems, Warren, NJ, USA) and the Strecker® stent (Boston Scientific Corporation, Watertown, MA, USA), are meshworks cut from a stainless steel tube or knitted from tantalum wire.[29,38,45] Being compressed on to a balloon, they are introduced into the tracheobronchial tree after prior dilatation of the stenosis; once set in place, they are expanded by inflation of the introducer balloon. Fixation to the tracheobronchial wall is achieved by the expanding pressure. After some time these stents may become totally embedded into the bronchial wall.[12] Their lumen is relatively small, ranging from 7 mm for bronchial stenting up to 14 mm for tracheal stenting, while the length ranges between 2 and 8 cm. No covered balloon-expandable stents are available.

Self-expanding devices derive their expanding force either from their geometric configuration or from a so-called memory effect of special alloys. Stents of the former type include the Gianturco stent (Cook Inc., Bloomington, IN, USA) and the Wallstent™ (Schneider, Minneapolis, MA, USA). The Gianturco stent is constructed of a very rigid steel wire arranged in a crown using a zigzag configuration. Once released from its compressed form by retraction of a retaining sheath from the introducer on which it is mounted, the stent unfolds to its maximum preset diameter, usually in the region of 20 mm. A covered version has recently become available; this is particularly useful in the treatment of tracheobronchial fistulae.

The Wallstent endoprosthesis has a much tighter meshwork, also made of stainless steel filaments arranged in a spiral pattern, which transmit its expanding force on to a considerably greater surface area. This type of stent is available in several models using a variety of delivery systems. Older models are delivered via a complicated delivery system, which was rather unreliable in delivering the stent in the correct position; the new model is easier to use, and more precise. The older was limited to a diameter of 14 mm, whereas the new one is available in diameters up to 25 mm. The new model is available in covered as well as uncovered versions.

The most recent development in stenting of the central airways is the nitinol prosthesis. Nitinol is a binary alloy of nickel and titanium, the physical properties of which were first discovered at the Naval Ordinance Laboratories (NOL) in Maryland, USA. After mechanical deformation, a wire made of this material regains its preset configuration at temperatures above 20°C.[25] For the construction of endoprostheses, the wires are knitted to form a meshwork. In the authors' experience, the diameter of these stents decreases in a physiological manner during coughing manoeuvres, and the devices do not transmit unphysiologically high pressures to the bronchial wall during re-expansion. Most of the authors' experience in tracheobronchial stenting is with this system. Recently, this type of stent has become available on an experimental basis in a version covered by a membrane, which allows its use in tracheobronchial fistulae. However, this covered model is not yet commercially available.

The stent is released by withdrawing a plastic sheath constraining the endoprosthesis. The stent begins to expand, and establishes contact with the surface of the tracheobronchial wall. The memory metal effect, which has been set a body temperature, compels the stent to assume its designated, preprogrammed size and shape. As a rule, it needs 5 minutes to do so. Any manipulation during this expansion process, particularly pulling or pushing forces on the stent, should be avoided as it can cause compression and deformation. Defects of this nature cannot be corrected. After 5 minutes the delivery catheter can be withdrawn. Any bleeding caused by expansion of the stent in the tumour tissue should be identified and treated immediately. The surface of the stent is designed not to impair the function of the cilia on bronchial endothelium. Although the device is relatively rigid, it still retains a certain residual flexibility. The prototype stent used most frequently by the authors measured up to 16 mm in diameter, with a length of 4–10 cm. Use in tracheo-oesophageal fistulae is not possible until the stent is available in a covered version. The uncovered stent permits additional treatment with radiotherapy or laser in patients with recurrent tumours or protruding granulation tissue.

Tracheobronchial stents are inserted under sedation or anaesthesia, following previous dilatation or laser therapy of the stenotic segment under X-ray and endoscopic control. Dilatation and stent implantation are preceded by precise CT measurement of the tracheal or bronchial lumen, and by antibiotic prophylaxis. In the subsequent follow-up period, endoscopic examinations are performed initially after 1 week and then at monthly intervals. In addition, examinations are carried out if obstructive symptoms recur. Lung function tests are also conducted in order to detect early signs of constriction.

Non-metallic stents

The Dumon stent consists of a silicone tube of varying lengths and diameters with external protrusions for fixation.[10] Implantation is possible only by use of a special rigid introducing bronchoscope under general anaesthesia. The recommended technique of blind introduction under fluoroscopic control is rather cumbersome, and the delivery system is comparatively expensive. Several modifications have been proposed, including use of a standard bronchoscope, either by folding the prosthesis into the scope itself, or by loading it partially on to the bronchoscope. The authors have constructed a simple pusher with a conically shaped end through which ventilation can be provided while the stent is safely placed under visual control.

Owing to their geometry, older versions of the Dumon stent frequently become obliterated by sticky secretions, usually during the early post-implantation period. Freitag has developed an advanced type of silicone prosthesis, the dynamic stent, in which the ventral part is enforced by metallic bands for stabilization while the dorsal part is elastic, similar to the membranous wall of the airways. This allows narrowing of the airway diameter during coughing, which results in a higher air velocity and better mucus clearance. Fixation is achieved by advancing the bifurcated distal end of the prosthesis into both main bronchi. Isolated stenosis of one main bronchus or upper trachea, near the subglottic region, should not be treated with this type of stent because a considerable part of the unaffected airway would also be covered by the stent.[33]

Indications

The indications for tracheobronchial stenting include all benign and malignant stenoses of the tracheobronchial system that are accompanied by severe respiratory insufficiency. It is initially irrelevant whether the condition is caused by a primary bronchial tumour gradually constricting the lumen, a tumour infiltrating the tracheobronchial system resulting in ingrowth blocking the lumen, or extrinsic tumour compression of the trachea or bronchus resulting in respiratory insufficiency. Benign stenoses in the tracheobronchial system should be considered on an individual basis. A conservative approach is appropriate because long-term results are not yet available.

Patients' details

Since 1989, the authors have treated 402 patients (171 female and 231 male) with 638 stents in the tracheobronchial system. The diameter of the implanted stents ranged between 8 and 14 mm in the main bronchus and between 10 and 25 mm in the trachea. The age of the patients ranged between 4 and 86 years (mean 62 years). All patients had severe respiratory insufficiency caused by malignant or benign narrowing of the respiratory tract. In 36% the stents were used in benign disease and in 64% they were used to manage malignant conditions. Of the patients with malignancy, 48% had a bronchial carcinoma, 10% malignant lymphoma and 6% metastases from unknown primaries. The benign lesions were caused by iatrogenic injury during intubation, long-term ventilation and tracheostomy. In this group the authors found combined granulomatous scars and chondromalacia in about 25%, isolated scar formation in 12% and tracheobronchomalacia in 6%. In 16% there was a coexistent oesophageal compression or tracheo-oesophageal fistula. Stenoses were present in the trachea in 55%, the main bronchi in 25%, segmental bronchi in 8% and the subglottic larynx in 12%. Prior to implantation about 80% of the tumours had been treated with laser, 30% with radiation therapy, 42% with systemic chemotherapy and 30% with partial lung resection. Of the benign strictures, 30% had been previously treated surgically, especially by reconstruction of the trachea in patients with tracheomalacia. In patients with tracheo-oesophageal fistulae, only covered stents or Dumon stents can be used.

Follow-up

Patients are followed up with lung function tests and bronchoscopy at 1, 2 and 4 weeks, and then every 3 months for a year. After that time patients are examined yearly unless symptoms recur. The frequent bronchoscopic examinations in the immediate post-implantation period help to detect hyperplastic granuloma as well as tumour ingrowth, so that early treatment can be instituted. Infections are treated with antibiotics. If there is resistant infection or stent deformation it may be necessary to remove the stent. Many patients with malignancy require additional treatment, such as combined endoluminal radiation and percutaneous radiation therapy.

Results

Of the 638 stents implanted in 402 patients, 45.45% were flexible Boston Scientific Inc., (BSI) nitinol stents, 16.6% nitinol Memotherm stents from Angiomed, 8.2% Tantalum stents, 11.75% Dumon stents, 15.80% Wallstent™, and 2.2% were other types of stent (including the Gianturco stent) (Table 7.1). In approximately 90%, stent implantation led to a significant improvement in respiratory function and diminution of symptoms. In nearly all cases there was sufficient improvement for patients to leave hospital. In malignant stenoses the median survival time was 5.4 months (range 8 hours–13 months). In more than 80%, death was caused by general progression of the disease. The median survival in patients with benign disease is 28 months (range 5–78 months).

Infections after implantation occurred in 44 out of 638 implantation procedures and were adequately treated with antibiotics. Twenty-nine deformed stents had to be removed because of deterioration of respiratory function. In 6 other cases deformed stents have been left *in situ* because respiratory function remained adequate and there were no clinical symptoms. Forty-two stent migrations have been observed. In 4 the stent displacement was significant and the device had to be removed. In 17% of all implanted stents, there was diminution of the stent lumen either by granulation tissue or tumour ingrowth (Table 7.1). Tumour overgrowth at the ends of covered or Dumon stents was treated by coaxial insertion of additional stents projecting beyond the new tumour growth, or by surgical resection. Laser therapy should not be undertaken within Dumon stents or plastic-covered metallic stents, as the plastic material forming the wall of these devices is flammable. Tantalum stents are prone to compression, especially in the trachea. Considerable pressures are generated within the thoracic cavity and the stent may collapse under the strain. This is especially true for the Strecker stent (Fig. 7.1), but can also occur with the Palmaz stent. If this occurs, it may be difficult, if not impossible, to remove the

Table 7.1

Comparison of complications experienced with implantation of various types of stents (n = 638) into 402 patients.

	Nitinol BSI stent	Nitinol Memotherm stent	Tantalum stent	Dumon's stent	Wallstent	Others (including the Gianturco stent)
No. of implanted stents (n = 638)	290	106	52	75	101	14
Complications						
Displacement	9 (3)	9 (8.6)	1 (2.7)	2 (2.7)	18 (17.4)	–
Infection	8 (2.8)	5 (5.1)	9 (16.6)	16 (22.2)	8 (7.9)	–
Deformation	3 (1)	2 (1.7)	18 (36)	0	6 (5.7)	–
Extraction	9 (3)	2 (1.7)	11 (21)	4 (5.5)	8 (7.9)	–
Tumour overgrowth	49 (14)	11 (10.3)	11 (21)	12 (16.7)	19 (19)	–
Total no. of complications	58 (20)	24 (24)	19 (38)	20 (27.8)	21 (21)	–

– data not available.
Figures in parentheses denote percentages.

(a)

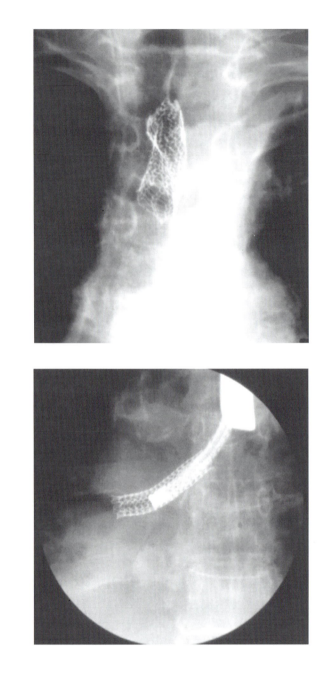

(b)

Figure 7.1
Different variants of the tantalum Strecker stent for implantation in the tracheobronchial system. (a) Torqued and deformed tantalum stent in the trachea. (b) With a diameter of 8 mm the stent in the right main bronchus is resistant enough against force from outside.

stent from the airways once it has been fully integrated into the bronchial wall. The use of a stronger tantalum wire for the knitted stent has not solved this problem. With both the Palmaz and Strecker stents, excessive formation of granulation tissue or tumour ingrowth can lead to restenosis or complete occlusion. Because of these problems, the authors do not recommend the application of these stents in the central airways.[2]

In the authors experience, use of the Gianturco stent is accompanied by significant problems: as the expanding pressure of this stent is concentrated on to a very small surface area, especially at the pointed ends, perforation of the bronchial wall is common, resulting in tracheobronchial fistula, or fatal haemorrhage due to erosion of the pulmonary artery. The Gianturco stent is fixed by hooks at the pointed ends and cannot be readily removed in case of complications. Moreover, the gaps between the wires are very large and early reocclusion by prolapsing tumour is comparatively frequent. In the authors' opinion, use of this device should be restricted to extrinsic tumour compression.[3] They have observed stress fractures of the struts of the stent, comparable to those of the Günther vena cava filter, with subsequent migration of these filaments into mediastinal strictures and the risk of perforation of the aorta, oesophagus or superior vena cava. Such fractures have been observed mainly in patients with benign disease who survived for a considerable time following implantation. The new improved Gianturco–Rösch variant avoids some of the disadvantages of the original Gianturco stent (Fig. 7.2). Remaining problems are related to the size of the introducer system and the tendency to migration of the covered version of the stent.

Figure 7.2
The Gianturco and Gianturco–Rösch stent. (a) The Gianturco stent. Lateral view after implantation of two conventional Gianturco stents in the trachea to treat a tracheomalacia. (b) The new covered Gianturco–Rösch stent for implantation in tracheo-oesophageal fistulae.

(a)

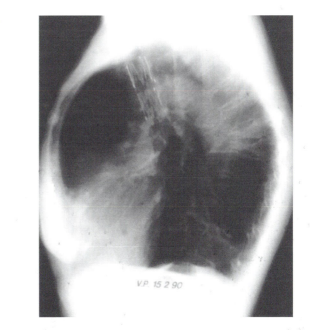

(b)

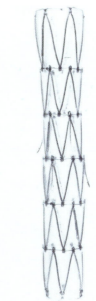

The Wallstent has a good expanding force and sufficient flexibility to allow secretion and expectoration of mucus during coughing, as well as a good epithelialization of the stent filaments. The major problems encountered with this stent in the past were related to the cumbersome delivery system which made it difficult to position the stent accurately. The new airways Wallstent is much easier to use. Despite its pointed edges, perforation does not occur. Tumour ingrowth and encroachment by granulation tissue do occur. However, removal of the stent can be difficult, and can be achieved only by destruction of the stent and extraction of filaments individually.[5] The covered version of the stent for use in tracheo-oesophageal fistulae is easy to position, but shows a tendency to migration in some cases, like other covered stents (Fig. 7.3).

The nitinol stent by Boston Scientific has adequate rigidity and flexibility due to its memory effect and its geometric configuration. Removal is possible in case of misplacement. Migration has not been observed, nor have there been any problems with the transport of secretions, expectoration of mucus, epithelialization of the

(a)

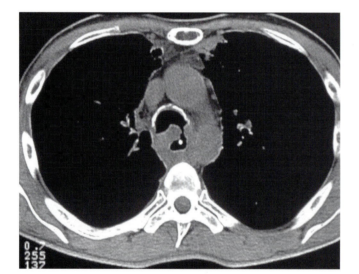

(b)

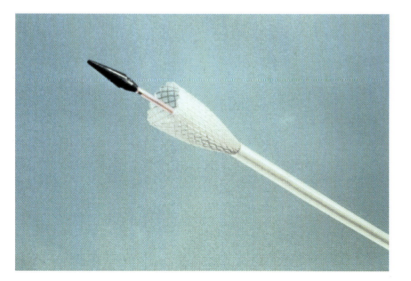

Figure 7.3
A 72-year-old woman with a tracheo-oesophageal fistula as complication of a perforating neoplasm of the bronchus. (a) CT shows tracheo-oesophageal fistula. (b) Covered Wallstent for the therapy of stenotic lesions with a concomitant tracheo-oesophageal fistula.

filaments or predisposition to infection. A major disadvantage was the absence of an acceptable delivery system for the original stent but this problem has now been rectified. A covered version of the stent is not yet commercially available (Fig. 7.4).

The nitinol Memotherm stent has a simple and easy to use delivery system (Fig. 7.5). The authors did not observe any significant infections after stent implantation. Tumour ingrowth leading to deterioration of respiratory function is best treated with endoscopic laser therapy. There was one case of mediastinal emphysema after placement of a nitinol Memotherm stent; the patient died within 24 hours. At post-mortem examination it was not possible to establish whether the emphysema had been caused by rupture of the tumour-infiltrated tracheal wall or by the application of laser immediately before stent implantation.

Implantation of the Dumon stent is performed under bronchoscopic guidance. The Dumon stent has certain disadvantages: as the flow of air inside the stent is slower than inside self-expanding stents, occlusion by secretions is comparatively

Figure 7.4
The flexible nitinol Becker stent from BSI. (a) Three BSI nitinol stents in tracheobronchomalacia placed by bronchoscopical control. (b) Covered nitinol stent for the therapy of stenotic lesions with tracheo-oesophageal fistulae.

(a)

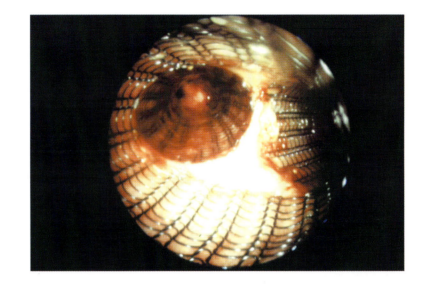

(b)

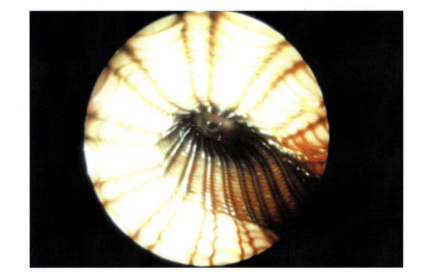

(a)

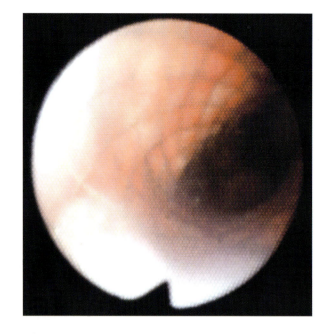

(b)

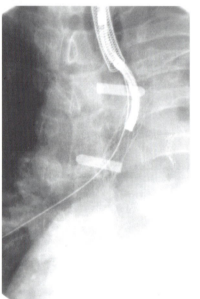

Figure 7.5
(a) Bronchoscopic view of a well-placed nitinol Memotherm stent crossing the bifurcation to the right main bronchus.
(b) Documentation of a placed Memotherm stent during concomitant endoscopic control.

frequent.[33] In smaller bronchi, the inner diameter of the stent is very small owing to the thickness of the plastic material, thus leaving very little lumen for ventilation and clearance of secretions. Stenting of the subglottic area and of very short stenoses is not recommended as secure fixation cannot be reliably accomplished. As the stent is plastic, laser cannot be used on tumour overgrowth. Surgical intervention to deal with problems following implantation is more common than with any other type of stent.

The authors have treated over 100 patients with tracheo-oesophageal fistulae with the use of covered BSI nitinol-type stents, the Gianturco–Rösch stents, Wallstent endoprotheses and Dumon stents, without significant complications (Fig. 7.6). However, covered stents are prone to migration.

Figure 7.6 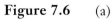 (a)

Covered stents are implanted more and more in the therapy of malignant and benign compression syndrome to the oesophagus and the trachea at the same time. In this case a 25 mm Wallstent has been implanted in the oesophagus and two 14 mm nitinol Memotherm stents have been implanted into the trachea. (a) CT shows both the intraluminal stents. (b) A lateral view of both stents.

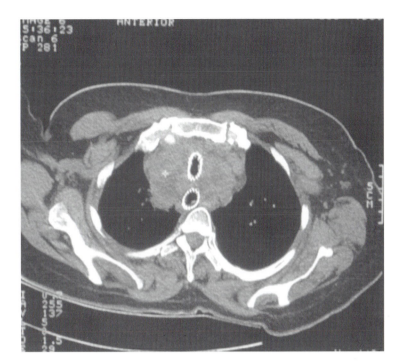

(b)

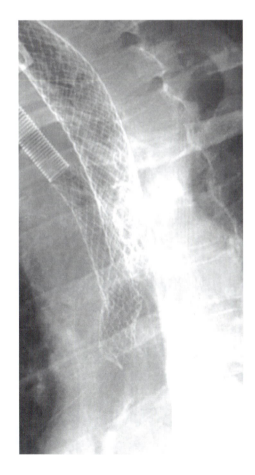

Conclusions

In contrast to surgery, radiation therapy[4,20,27,35] or laser therapy,[21] balloon dilatation[7] leads to a rapid improvement of respiratory function after treatment of malignant or benign bronchial stenoses. Unfortunately, this improvement is often short-lasting because of reobstruction caused by tumour ingrowth or overgrowth, tracheomalacia or growth of granulation tissue. Bronchial patency can be prolonged by combining treatment modalities. In 1966, Montgomery was the first to describe the use of a T-tube to keep open the tracheal lumen.[34] Several reports on the use of internal and external rigid prostheses followed,[1,8–10,36,37,53] before Wallace and co-workers published their results using a self-expanding stent in the therapy of tracheobronchial stenoses.[51] Following the initial report in 1987, the present authors begin to use the Gianturco Z-stent. In one case of a benign stenosis, the trachea remains patent 8 years after implantation. There have been several reports on the use of the Gianturco Z-stent in tracheobronchial stenoses.[40,43,48,49]

The high risk of perforation that is associated with the use of the Gianturco stent[42] led the authors to abandon its use in 1989 in favour of a modified Strecker stent made from tantalum. This stent is easy to use but has an inadequate expanding force compared with other types of stent.[6,11,45,48] The degree of deformation increases in proportion to the diameter of the stent. Although this does not usually lead to decreased ventilation, the relatively frequent deformation of the stent limits its use in the trachea. Implantation of this stent should be reserved for bronchial stenoses.[41]

The Palmaz stent is not suitable for implantation in the tracheobronchial system. It is too rigid, prone to collapse, too short, and has an inadequate calibre.[5,6]

The Gianturco–Rösch stent is less prone to stress fractures of the struts because of a change in design and manufacturing. Its delivery system is large but easy to handle. Like the Wallstent and the BSI nitinol stent, this stent is available in a covered version for implantation in tracheo-oesophageal fistulae.

Delivery of the Wallstent has been made easier by the development of a redesigned delivery system that allows implantation of stents with diameters of up to 25 mm. The sharp ends of the metallic stent filaments remain a problem which should be addressed.

The replacement of tantalum by nitinol in the Strecker stent has led to markedly improved rigidity.[24] This type of stent is commercially available as the Becker stent; only an uncovered version is available so far. The delivery system requires significant improvement.

The nitinol Memotherm stent combines adequate flexibility with rigidity. However, this rigid device cannot easily be removed in cases of misplacement.

The Dumon stent has expensive storage requirements because of the need to keep in stock a large variety of different elements of the implantation system. It also impairs elimination of secretions and expectoration of mucus, leading to retention of secretions and occasionally to infection. In order to minimize the lack of flexibility during respiration and coughing, the manufacturer has improved the stent design by modelling the device on the anatomy of the trachea in combining rigid front and sides with a flexible dorsal segment that allows variation in calibre during breathing (Freitag stent).

The plastic covering of stents of any type increases the retention of secretions, which can lead to infection. However, the use of plastic-covered endoprostheses is mandatory in the management of tracheobronchial fistulae. In addition, the plastic covering protects the stent lumen from early tumour ingrowth and invasion by granulation tissue. However, granulation tissue can still grow at the ends of the stent and may lead to restenosis, requiring treatment with either surgery or the insertion of an overlapping stent. Laser cannot be used because of the risk of setting fire to the plastic material.

In summary, stent insertion represents an attractive alternative to surgery or repeated laser therapy in the management of tracheobronchial stenoses. The median survival of patients with malignant or benign strictures treated with stents is comparable to surgery and superior to balloon dilatation, laser treatment and radiotherapy. Tracheo-oesophageal fistulae can be managed with covered stents. These are sometimes combined with oesophageal stent insertion. Stenting leads to a rapid improvement in symptoms, improving the quality of life and often allowing the patient to resume normal activity.

References

1   Andersen HC, Egknud P. Intratracheal tube treatment of stenosis of the trachea. *Acta Otolaryngol* 1967; **224**: 29–30.
2   Becker HC, van Bodegom K. Der Einsatz des Strecker-Stents in der Trachea. In: Kollath J, Liermann D (eds) *Stents II*. Konstanz: Schnetztor-Verlag, 1992; **2**: 216–225.
3   Becker HD, Wagner B, Liermann D, Urhoij S, Mechmann S. Stenting of the central airways. In: Liermann D (ed.) *Stents*. Poly Science Montreal, 1995; **11.2**: 249–255.
4   Böttger T, Ungeheuer E. Benigne und semimaligne Bronchustumoren. *Dtsch Ärzteblatt* 1987; **84**: 2398–2404.
5   Bohndorf K, Günther RW, Huerter T, Kurzewa D, Vorwerk D. Use of a metallic self-expandable stent in the tracheobronchial system: first clinical experiences. *Radiology* 1990; **177**: 297.
6   Bohndorf K, Kurzeja A, Schlöndorff G, Vorwerk D, Günther W. Implantation selbstexpandierender endoprothesen (Wallstent) bei benignen trachealobstruktionen. In: Kollath J, Liermann D (eds) *Stents II*. Konstanz: Schnetztor-Verlag, 1992; S234–242.
7   Cohen MD, Weber TR, Rao CC. Balloon dilatation of tracheal and bronchial stenosis. *Am J Radiol* 1984; **142**: 477–478.
8   Cohen RC, Filler RM, Konuma K, Bahoric A, Knet G. Smith C. A new model of tracheal stenosis and its repair with free periosteal grafts. *J Thorac Cardiovasc Surg* 1986; **92**: 296–304.
9   Do YS, Song HY, Lee HL *et al.* Esophagorespiratory fistula associated with esophageal cancer: treatment with a Gianturco stent tube. *Radiology* 1993; **187**: 673–677.
10 Dumon JF. A dedicated tracheobronchial stent. *Chest* 1990; **97**: 328–332.
11 Fallone BG, Wallace DS, Gianturco C. Elastic characteristics of the self-expanding metallic stents. *Invest Radiol* 1988; **23**: 370–376.
12 Grewe P, Krampe K, Müller KM, Becker HD. Macroscopic and histomorphologic alterations of the bronchial wall after implantation of nitinol stents. In Liermann D (ed.) *Stents*. Poly Science Montreal, 1995; **11.2**: 256–259.
13 Grillo HC. Tracheal surgery. *Scand J Cardiovasc Surg* 1983; **17**: 67–77.
14 Hagel KJ, Rautenberg HW. Ballondilatation bei angeborenen Pulmonalstenosen im Kindesalter. *Herz/Kreislauf* 1987; **19**: 343–347.
15 Hajek M. Rekonstruktive Operationen bei Trachealstenosen und erworbenen Tracheo-Oesophagealfisteln. *Z Erkr Atmungsorgane* 1986; **166**: 116–118.
16 Hartmann CA, Mollinedo J. Pathologisch-anatomische Gesichtspunkte seltener Bronchustumoren. *Prax Pneumol* 1981; **35**: 735–736.
17 Hartung W. Pathologie der Lungenfehlbildung. *Thoraxchirurgie* 1975; **23**: 194.
18 Hecker W. *Elementare Kinderchirurgie*. München: Urban & Schwarzenberg, 1975.
19 Helbig D. *Chirurgische Pädiatrie*. Stuttgart: Schattauer, 1974
20 Herzog H, Heitz M, Keller R, Graedel E. Surgical therapy for expiratory collapse of the trachea and large bronchi. In: Grilo H, Eschapasse H (eds) *International trends in general thoracic surgery. Major challenges*, vol 2. Philadelphia: Saunders, 1987.
21 Hetzel MR, Nixon C, Edmonstone WM. Lasertherapy in 100 tracheobronchial tumors. *J Thorax* 1985; **40**: 341–345.
22 Ilberg CV. 7 Jahre Erfahrung mit der Tracheaquerresektion. *Laryngl Rhinol Otol* 1985; **64**: 40–42.

23 Ivemark B. *Kinder-Pathologie*. Berlin: Springer, 1974

24 Johnston MR, Loeber N, Hilleyer P, Stephenson LW, Edmunds LH. External stent for repair of secondary tracheomalacia. *Ann Thorac Surg* 1980; **30**: 291–296.

25 Kauffmann GB, Mayo I. The metal with a memory. *Invent Technol* 1993; 18–23.

26 Kloos K, Vogel M. *Pathologie der Perinatalperiode*. Stuttgart: Thieme, 1974.

27 Krumhaar D. Neoplasmen des Mediastinums. In: Trendelenburg F (ed.) *Handbuch der Inneren Medizin*, Bd.IV.B Berlin: Springer, 1985; 582–651.

28 Kunz H. *Operationen im Kindesalter*. Stuttgart: Thieme, 1973.

29 Liermann D. Lörcher U, Rauber K *et al.* Stents in the tracheobronchial system – first results. *Eur Radiol* 1991; **1304**: 55.

30 Liermann D, Rust M. First experiences with a new memory metallic endoprosthesis in the tracheobrochial system. In: Liermann D (ed.) *Stents*. Poly Science Montreal, 1995; **11.2**: 260–265.

31 Maaßen W. Thorakoskopie: Chirugische Technik. *Pneumologie* 1989; **43**: 53–54.

32 Martini N, Goodner TJ. Di Angielo GJ, Beatti EJ. Tracheo-oesophageal fistula due to cancer. *J Thorac Cardiovasc Surg* 1970; **59**: 319.

33 Miyazawa T, Doi M, Mineshita M, Kurata T, Suei T, Yamakido M. The placement of the Dumon stent for airway stenosis. *J Jap Soc Bronchol* 1993; **15**: 749–756.

34 Montgomery WW. T-tube tracheal stent. *Arch Otolaryngol* 1965; **82**: 320–321.

35 Morr H. Tumoren. In: Fabel H (ed.) *Pneumologie*. München: Urban & Schwarzenberg, 1989; 391–426.

36 Neville WE, Bolanowski PJP, Soltanzadeh H. Prosthetic reconstruction of the trachea and the carina. *J Thorac Cardiovasc Surg* 1982; **83**: 414–417.

37 Nissen R. Tracheaplastik zur Beseitigung der Erschlaffung der Pars membranacea. *Schweiz Med Wochenschr* 1954; **84**: 219.

38 Palmaz JC. Intravascular stents. In: Kollath J, Liermann D (eds) *Stents II*. Konstanz: Schnetztor-Verlag, 1992; S162–173.

39 Rauber K, Kronenberger H. Perorale transluminale Dilatation maligner Bronchusverschlüsse. *Fortschr Röntgenstr* 1987; **147**: 261–265.

40 Rauber K, Franke C, Rau WS. Self-expanding stainless steel endotracheal stents: an animal study. *J Cardiovasc Intervent Radiol* 1989; **12**: 274.

41 Rauber K, Franke CH, Seyed Ali S, Bensmann G. Experimentelle Erfahrungen mit Nitinol-Prothesen. In: Kollath J, Liermann D (eds) *Stents – Ein aktueller Überblick*. Konstanz: Schnetztor-Verlag, 1990; 1: 65–70.

42 Rauber K, Franke C, Rau WS, Syed-Ali A. Venendurchwanderung bei Gianturco–Wallace-Stents. Zentralblatt d Radiol,- Radiology, 1990; 141.3-4: 293.

43 Rauber K, Weimar B, Hofmann M, Rau WS. Clinical experiences with endotracheal Gianturco Z stents. *Eur Radiol* 1991; **1**: 56.

44 Rehbein F. *Kinderchirugische Operationen*. Stuttgart: Hippokrates, 1976.

45 Richter GM. Theoretische Grundlagen des ballonexpandierbaren Palmaz Stents. In: Kollath J, Liermann D (eds) *Stents – Ein aktueller Überblick*, Konstanz: Schnetztor-Verlag, 1990; **1**: 50–57.

46 Sandritter W, Thomas C. *Histopathologie*. Stuttgart: Schattauer, 1977

47 Sandritter W, Thomas C. *Makropathologie*. Stuttgart: Schattauer, 1977

48 Sawada S, Fujiwara Y, Koyama T *et al.* Clinical experience with expandable metallic stent placement for treatment of tracheal and bronchial stenosis. *Radiology* 1990; **177**: 297.

49 Simonds AK, Irving JD, Clarke SW, Dick R. Use of expandable metal stents in the treatment of bronchial obstruction. *J Thorax* 1989; **44**: 680–681.

50 Vollmar J. Konnatale Mißbildungen der Arterien: Coarctatio aortae. In: Vollmar J (ed.) *Kompendium der Gefäßchirugie*. Stuttgart: Thieme, 1986; 76–88.

51 Wallace MJ, Charsangagevej C, Ogawa K *et al.* Tracheobronchial tree: expandable metallic stents used in experimental and clinical applications. *Radiology* 1986; **26**: 309.

52 Weerda H, Zöllner C, Schlenter W. Die Behandlung der Stenosen des laryngo-trachealen Übergangs und der cervikalen Trachea. *HNO* 1986; **34**: 156–161.

53 Westaby S, Jackson JW. A bifurcated silicone rubber stent for relief of tracheo-bronchial obstructions. *J Thorac Cardiovasc Surg* 1982; **83**: 414–417.

54 Windorfer A, Stephan U. *Mucoviscidose,-Cystische Fibrose*. Stuttgart: Thieme Verlag, 1968.

55 Wissler H. *Erkrankungen der Lungen und Bronchien im Kindesalter*. Stuttgart: Thieme Verlag, 1972.

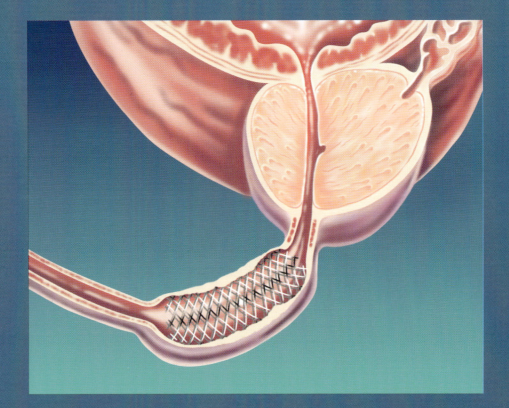

Chapter 8
Metal stents in the urinary tract

D. Rickards and E.J.G. Milroy

Introduction

Metal stents were first used in the urinary tract in the treatment of recurrent strictures in the bulbar membranous urethra in 1985. The Wallstent™ (Schneider, Minneapolis, MN, USA) was originally developed for endovascular use in recurrent arterial stenoses following balloon angioplasty.[1] After experimental use of this stent in dogs, early reports on 8 patients in whom the stent had been used in the urethra suggested that such devices might have a significant role in the treatment of recurrent urethral strictures.[2] Subsequently, the use of this stent has been extended for the treatment of prostatic outflow obstruction attributable to both benign and malignant disease and in the treatment of urethral strictures. The metal stents can be either temporary or permanent, the principal difference between the two types being that the former are intraluminal, will encrust with phosphatic debris if left long enough in contact with urine, and so are liable to become infected. A permanent stent becomes covered with urothelium, thereby excluding it from contact with urine and avoiding the risks of infection, encrustation and stent migration. Both types are used in the treatment of bladder outflow obstruction and urethral stricture; they are also beginning to be used in cases of ureteric stricture, but no long-term results are yet available. Biodegradable stents are now being tried on an experimental basis.

Metal stents in the treatment of urethral stricture

Urethral stricture is a common clinical urological problem that can occur at any age and should be suspected in men under 50 years of age who develop outflow obstruction, specifically if there is a history of perineal trauma, urethritis or instrumentation. Strictures do not usually become clinically apparent until the calibre of the urethral lumen is less than 3 mm.

Attempts to treat urethral strictures can be traced back for several centuries, but John Hunter in the 18th century produced the first detailed study.[3] Urethral dilatation was, for many years, the only therapeutic modality until the introduction of urethrotomy by Civiali,[4] using a urethrotome that with subsequent modifications, included the attachment of a cutting blade to a filiform guide. Otis, in 1872, produced a specifically designed instrument still in use today.[5] Urethral dilatation has been largely replaced by endoscopic urethrotomy, the cure rates following such treatment varying between 25 and 90% in a large series (mean 64%).[6] Konnak and Kogan[7] reported a 58% recurrence rate within 6 months with an additional 33% beyond 1 year. It is accepted that, after a second urethrotomy, this operation is associated with a considerably reduced rate of success. Recently, the combined use of urethrotomy followed by intermittent self-catheterization has been described.[8] However, although this procedure is effective, it is often unacceptable to the patient. In the event of failure of these therapies, or when patient compliance is affected, until recently the only therapeutic option was that of reconstructive urethroplasty. Reconstructive surgery produces good results with traumatic stricture but is less effective in cases of iatrogenic or infective strictures.

The aim of these procedures is to replace damaged fibrotic urothelium with revascularized urothelium. In dilatation and urethrotomy, the fibrotic band forming the stricture is disrupted in the hope that it will heal by the ingrowth of new urothelium without restenosis. Long-term or intermittent self-catheterization is aimed at maintaining the calibre of the urethral lumen while this healing takes place. Metal stents represent a new approach to the treatment of recurrent urethral stricture: they hold open a previously dilated stricture while it becomes covered with new urothelium, which will then prevent restenosis of the urethra. Temporary stents that do not become covered with urothelium have also been described recently.[9] These are left within the dilated stricture for a month, to allow for the ingrowth of urothelium outside the stent. Although these stents avoid the use of a permanent implant, they tend to migrate, and also become encrusted because of their contact with urine. Results with permanently implanted stents, from the Middlesex Hospital and from Professor J. P. Sarramon's unit in France (the centres that jointly pioneered the technique), are encouraging.[10]

Permanent stents available for the treatment of urethral stricture

The first stent used was a modification of the Wallstent for endovascular use that is now known as the Urolume™ Wallstent (American Medical Systems, Minnetonka, MN, USA). The use of a modified Strecker stent (Boston Scientific Corporation, Watertown, MA, USA) in the canine urethra has been described.[11] This is a modified endovascular stent knitted from a single tantalum wire, which becomes completely covered with epithelium by 6 months. A nitinol (nickel–titanium alloy) Strecker stent knitted from a single wire has also been used in 18 normal canine urethras to study the degree of epithelial covering.[12]

Temporary stents in urethral stricture

The use of temporary stents (which do not become covered with epithelium) in the treatment of prostatic outflow obstruction has led to their use in cases of urethral stricture. The Urocoil™ (Fig. 8.1) is a nickel–titanium coil that is placed in a dilated urethral stricture. The device comes in lengths of 4–8 cm and is mounted on a catheter (Fig. 8.2) which, when released, holds the urethral open to a calibre of between 8 and 10 mm. It has an undulating shape, intended to maintain the position of the stent within the urethra;[13,14] nevertheless, migration is a problem (Fig. 8.3). The Urocoil-S™ has an anchoring section that is connected to the urethral stent via a single helical transsphincteric spacer that permits sphincter closure and is intended to prevent migration (Fig. 8.4 and Fig. 8.5). These devices can be left within the urethra for up to 1 year and produce very few complications while in place; however, displacement remains a significant problem. Repositioning is usually not difficult. The stent is implanted

Figure 8.1
Plain film of the Urocoil deployed within the proximal anterior urethra (arrow). Its undulating shape should maintain its position within the urethra.

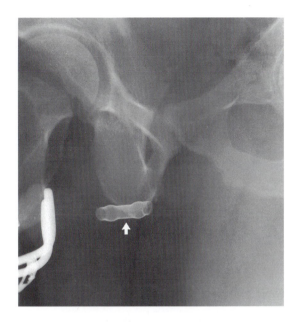

Figure 8.2
The Urocoil premounted on its delivery catheter.

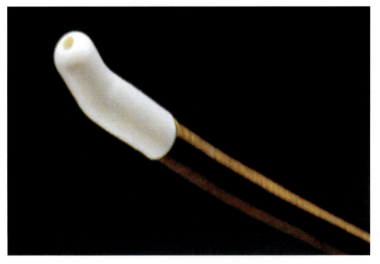

Figure 8.3
Ascending urethrogram showing a Urocoil that has migrated distally, having been placed initially across a tight stricture (arrow). The stent was easily repositioned.

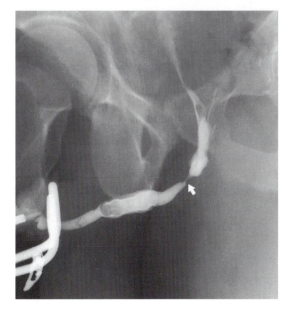

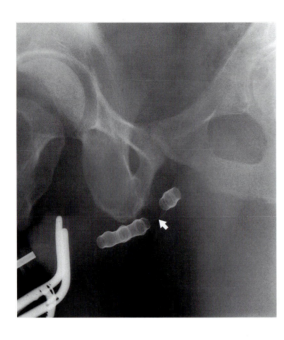

Figure 8.4
The Urocoil-S has a transsphincteric wire (arrow). The proximal smaller coil lies above the distal sphincter and stabilizes the longer coil in the anterior and bulbar urethra.

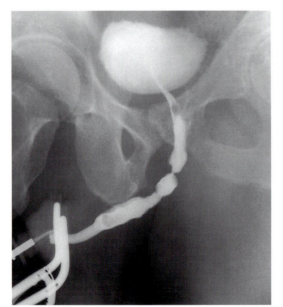

Figure 8.5
Ascending urethrogram showing the Urocoil-S in situ.

under radiographic control. It can be removed by grasping the end of the coil at urethroscopy; as this is pulled out of the urethra, the coil unravels. The flexibility and smoothness of the Urocoil system allow it to be used along the entire length of the urethra, giving it an advantage over permanent urethral stents. Use of these stents is aimed at holding open, for a limited period, a stricture that has either been dilated or subjected to urethrotomy, thus allowing healing and fibrosis to stabilize without the occurrence of long-term restenosis. The ideal device would be an absorbable or biodegradable stent and such devices are being introduced by a Finnish group.[15] Experiments in animals have shown that such stents, made of reinforced poly-l-lactide, when implanted into animal urethras become covered with epithelium by 6 months; by 12 months they are macroscopically degraded, with only a slight inflammatory reaction at the site of the stent.

Urolume stent for urethral stricture

The greatest experience, among all types of stents, has been with the permanent Urolume Wallstent. This is a woven, self-expanding, tubular mesh of fine super-alloy wire available in lengths of 2 and 3 cm, with maximum diameter of 14 mm (42 Fr) (the lengths and diameters stated refer to the unconstrained measurements of the stent). The expansile force of the mesh holds the stent against the walls of the urethra, allowing urothelium to grow over and through the implanted material. Should the stent not fully deploy within the strictured area, it will not achieve its final diameter and will be longer than its stated length. The extent to which the stent opens depends on the degree of dilatation of the stricture before deployment of the stent, and on the compliance of the particular stricture.

The Urolume stent is commercially available on a delivery system (Fig. 8.6) that holds the stent in place by two catches: releasing the first catch allows the protective sheath to be partially withdrawn; complete deployment of the stent requires release of the second catch.

Indications
Only strictures in the bulbar urethra are suitable for stenting. Stents placed within the pendulous penile urethra in a patient who is sexually active may cause pain during erection as the area of urethra that is stented will not elongate. Permanent stents should not be used in strictures following urethroplasty or pelvic fracture stricture: in these cases there is a high risk of fibrous tissue growing through the stent and causing significant intrastent restricturing. Those strictures that involve the distal sphincter mechanism, often as a result of transurethral resection of the prostate gland (TURP), can be stented in combination with an artificial urinary sphincter distal to the sphincter stricture (Fig. 8.7).

Figure 8.6
The Urolume stent and the insertion device.

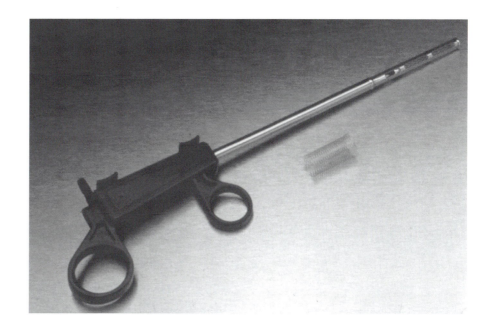

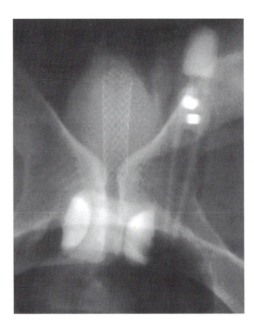

Figure 8.7
A Urolume has been placed across a sphincter stricture following TURP. A Brantley–Scott prosthesis has been placed around the proximal posterior urethra to maintain continence.

Preoperative imaging
A good-quality ascending and descending urethrogram is essential to identify the exact position and length of the stricture (Fig. 8.8). The proximity of the stricture to the active area of the distal sphincter is best demonstrated during interruption of micturition in a descending study.[16]

Urolume stent insertion in cases of urethral stricture
Stents are usually inserted under general anaesthesia, but local or regional anaesthesia can be used if the stricture is easy to dilate. Initially, the stricture is dilated up to 10 mm using bougies. However, if the stricture is very narrow or

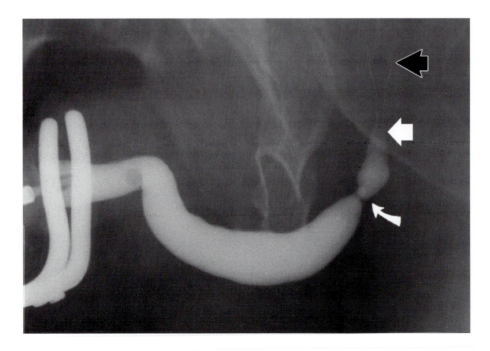

Figure 8.8
Ascending urethrogram prior to stent insertion. The stricture (curved arrow) is in the bulbar urethra. The distal aspect of the distal sphincter mechanism (arrow) and the verumontanum are well seen on ascending studies.

fibrosed, optical urethrotomy is performed. It is important to make two or three radial cuts to ensure that, when the stent is implanted, it lies centrally within the urethral lumen; a single cut can result in the stent lying eccentrically.

The length of the strictured urethra is assessed from the preoperative urethrogram and endoscopic measurement. The correct length of stent, either 2 or 3 cm, preloaded on its delivery system, is then selected; this should extend at least 0.5 cm beyond the strictured area into normal urethra. A standard 0° telescope is inserted down the centre of the delivery system, which is introduced into the urethra. Release of the first safety catch allows the outer sheath of the delivery system to be withdrawn to the second safety position as the stent expands, shortening into the urethra, before its final release. The position of the stent within the strictured area can be checked by sliding the telescope up and down the length of the stent. Precise positioning of the stent, before its release from the delivery system, is vital to prevent recurrent stricture formation, which would inevitably occur if the entire stricture were not covered by the stent. It is important not to allow the stent to encroach upon the sphincter active area, as this can result in incontinence. Following insertion, the stents become completely covered with urothelium. In most patients, this occurs within the first 1–3 months after implantation, although in some patients it may take up to 6–9 months, particularly in cases of posturethroplasty stricture (for which the stent is not recommended). In the first 4–6 weeks after implantation a variable hyperplastic reaction occurs as the urothelium grows over the wires of the stent. This is commonly seen in cases of posturethroplasty stricture, presumably because of the presence of squamous rather than normal urethral epithelium. In all patients this hyperplastic reaction settles spontaneously within 6–12 months.

Postoperative assessment

In the first month following insertion, ascending urethrography shows somewhat irregular narrowing of the intrastent lumen, the diameter of which is reduced by between 16 and 100% of the stent diameter (Fig. 8.9 and Fig. 8.10).[16] Despite this attenuation of the intrastent lumen, contrast flows with unexpected ease

Figure 8.9

Ascending urethrogram 2 months after insertion of a Urolume across a bulbar stricture. There is irregularity of the intrastent lumen due to hyperplasia.

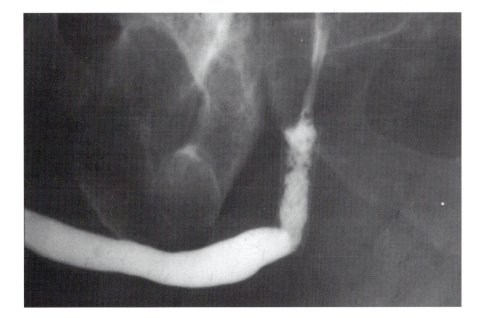

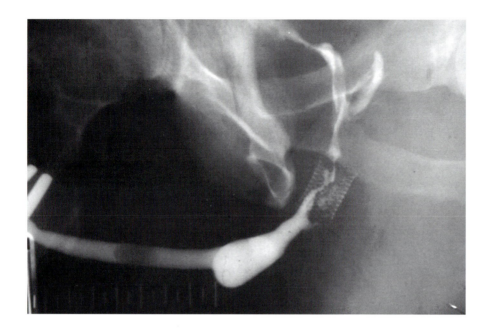

Figure 8.10
Ascending urethrogram 2 months after insertion of a Urolume for recurrent stricture following urethroplasty. There is marked narrowing of the intrastent lumen due to hyperplasia.

through the stent into the bladder. If endoscopy is performed at the same time, a hyperplastic urothelial reaction is identified, through which the endoscope passes easily. In most patients, urethrography at 6 months shows a smooth intrastent lumen, with excellent urothelial coating of the stent (Fig. 8.11). Urethroscopy at this stage shows a normal urothelium and it is difficult to identify the position of the stent.

Complications of urethral stents in cases of stricture

Incontinence
Stenting a stricture too close to the distal sphincter compromises sphincter function and can result in incontinence. Should this occur, it can be treated by the

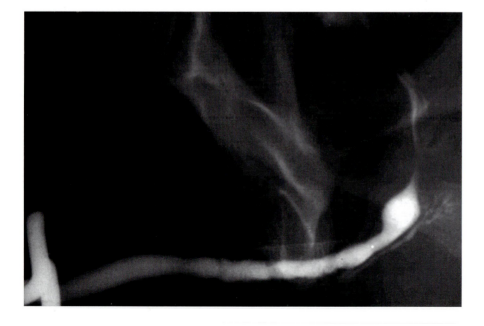

Figure 8.11
Ascending urethrogram 3 years following insertion of a Urolume. The intrastent lumen is adequate and the urothelial covering of the stent uniform and smooth. Despite the urothelial covering of the stent, a duct remains open.

insertion of an artificial urinary sphincter. This complication is most likely to occur in those patients who have sphincter strictures following TURP and insertion of both stent and artificial sphincter is an excellent therapeutic option (Fig. 8.7).

Post-micturition dribbling
Most patients with urethral stents complain of post-micturition dribbling of urine for 4–6 weeks after insertion. This is caused by urine remaining within the intrastent lumen on completion of micturition (Fig. 8.12); the stent holds the urethra open at all times and cannot collapse. This complication is exacerbated by an inflammatory exudate from reactive hyperplasia, seen within the first few weeks after insertion of the stent, although this improves spontaneously. However, 15–20% of patients report persistence of a minor degree of post-micturition dribbling.[17] Patients may also experience some mild discomfort at the site of the stent for the first 4–6 weeks following insertion. As previously mentioned, pain is felt during erection if the stent encroaches upon the penile urethra, but this usually settles spontaneously.

Haemospermia and water semen
A few patients will notice some bleeding during intercourse and they should be warned to avoid sexual intercourse for 2–3 weeks following insertion of the stent. Seminal fluid can also be a little more watery than usual because of dilution by a small amount of urine held within the stent after micturition. This has no clinical significance, but patients need to be warned about it before the procedure.

Intrastent hyperplasia
For the first 2–3 months after insertion, some patients complain of reduced flow rates and discomfort at the site of the stent. This is due to hyperplasia encroaching upon the intrastent lumen and is more common following

Figure 8.12
Descending urethrogram on interruption of micturition. Contrast remains within the Urolume; this residual urine will cause incontinence and dilution of semen.

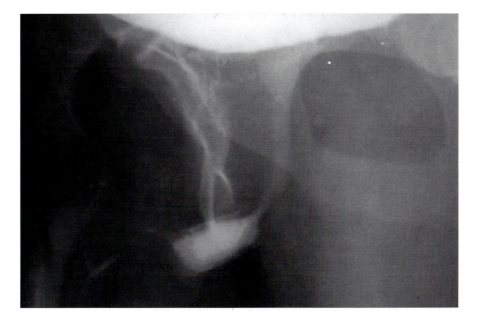

urethroplasty strictures. The hyperplasia can be resected endoscopically, but eventually settles spontaneously.

Restricturing
Development of fibrous tissue within the stent of the lumen is more commonly seen in patients following urethroplasty stricture (Fig. 8.13 and Fig. 8.14). Strictures just proximal or distal to the stent may be caused by inadequate

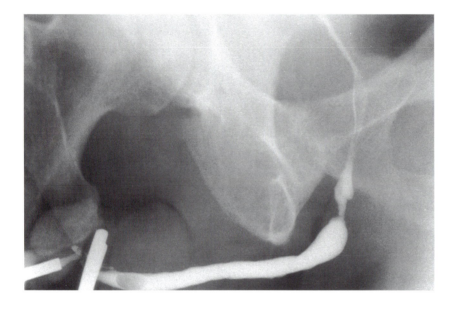
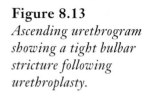

Figure 8.13
Ascending urethrogram showing a tight bulbar stricture following urethroplasty.

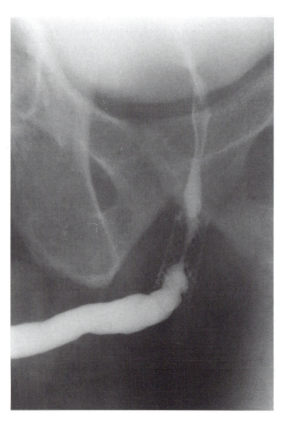

Figure 8.14
Ascending urethrogram 6 months after Urolume insertion into a post-urethroplasty stricture. There is an intrastent recurrent stricture.

covering of the original stricture (Fig. 8.15). A second, overlapping, stent is required to treat such strictures (Fig. 8.16).

Figure 8.15
Ascending urethrogram 2 years after stent insertion. There is a stricture just distal to the stent (arrow), which represents a stricture not covered at the original insertion.

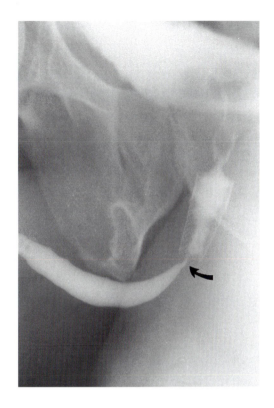

Figure 8.16
Ascending urethrogram 1 year after insertion of a second overlapping stent. There is excellent urothelial covering and no stricture.

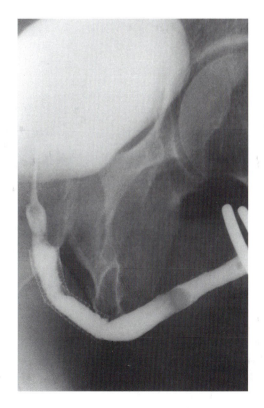

Stent removal

A poorly positioned stent can easily be removed soon after initial insertion. However, once the stent is fully covered with urothelium it is not possible to remove it endoscopically. Removal of the stent *en bloc* with end-to-end anastomosis is then the only therapeutic option.

Calculus formation

If the stent is not completely covered by urothelium, stones may form on the exposed wires (Fig. 8.17). These can cause obstruction or infection, any may pass spontaneously.

Long-term results following Urolume insertion for recurrent urethral stricture

Following the initial report by Milroy and colleagues in 1988,[18] many series have demonstrated the successful use of permanent stents in urethral stricture.[19,20] In 1995, Milroy and Allen reported long-term results with 50 patients, 27 of whom were followed up for at least 5 years.[21] Of these patients, 91% were satisfied with the stent, and 63% had no recurrence at endoscopy. Nine patients had recurrent stricture at either end of the stent; all were satisfactorily treated with an overlapping stent. It is almost certain that this complication was caused by slight misplacement of the original stent. Eight patients showed true intrastent narrowing; these can be regarded as cases of true failure of the technique because of a dense fibrosis that developed within the stent at the site of the original stricture (Fig. 8.18). This complication occurred in 2 of the 4 cases of post-traumatic urethral stricture that were treated in this series, and in 4 of the 8 cases of urethroplasty failure strictures after penile or scrotal inlay urethroplasty. True intrastent fibrosis also occurred after treatment in 1 of the 6 cases of infected stricture and in 1 of the 15 cases of catheter stricture. The long-term results of the Urolume stent in the treatment of recurrent stricture thus appear to be promising, but the technique is not suitable for all types of stricture and care

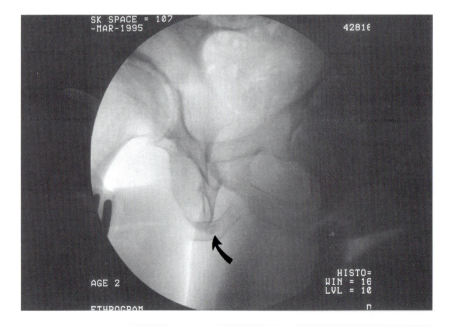

Figure 8.17
Plain film 5 years after Urolume stent insertion. A small stone has formed on uncovered wires (arrow). The patient passed this stone spontaneously.

Figure 8.18
Ascending urethrogram showing a tight intrastent stricture following stenting for a posturethroplasty stricture.

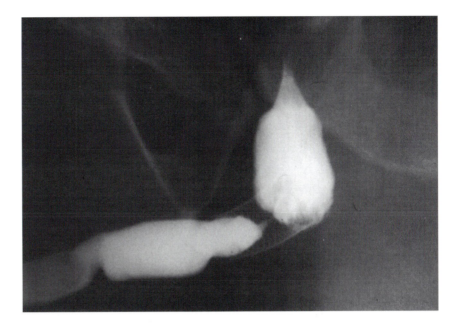

should be taken to avoid stenting those chronic strictures associated with extensive periurethral fibrosis. An Italian multicentre study reported the results with 76 unselected cases of stricture, with patients being followed up for between 1 and 14 months – in 29 cases for more than 1 year. Good relief of obstruction was obtained, but a 14% stricture recurrence rate was noted; however, only 3 patients had strictures within the lumen of the stent. Cystocopy at 1 year showed complete urothelial covering in 93% of cases. Interestingly, the authors found no correlation between stricture aetiology and postoperative problems, but stress the importance of implanting the stent in exactly the right position.[22]

Metal stents in dyssynergic sphincters

Patients with spinal cord injuries develop detrusor hyper-reflexia, which is associated with external striated sphincter dyssynergia (Fig. 8.19). Voiding depends upon adequate spontaneous relaxation of the external striated sphincter when autonomic bladder contractions occur. When high intravesical pressures occur because of sphincter dyssynergia, bladder pressures can be reduced by anticholinergic agents; satisfactory bladder emptying can be achieved by intermittent catheterization, chronic indwelling catheterization, external sphincterotomy or pharmacological therapy. Urinary diversion is an option. The complications of detrusor sphincter dyssynergia include vesico-ureteric reflux, urinary tract infection and renal insufficiency progressing to renal failure. Chronic catheterization is associated with the development of squamous cell metaplasia and 5% of patients develop cell carcinoma.

Treatment options

Endoscopic sphincterotomy is the procedure of choice, unless intermittent self-catheterization is appropriate or an anterior sacral route stimulator or is suitable. Even a properly performed single sphincterotomy may not achieve adequate

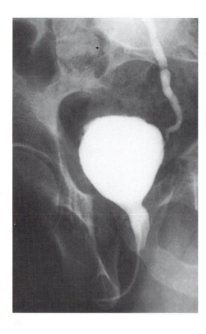

Figure 8.19
Cystogram demonstrating an open bladder neck, vesico-ureteric reflux and filling of the posterior urethra down to a dyssynergic distal sphincter.

bladder emptying, either because the sphincterotomy heals or because high pressures are developed by the pelvic floor. Even multiple sphincterotomies may prove ineffective. The use of a metal stent across the distal sphincter is an attractive alternative. The stent is placed over the distal sphincter under direct vision: in fertile patients, the stent is placed just up to the verumontanum, leaving the ejaculatory ducts uncovered; where fertility is not a consideration, the stent is placed well over the verumontanum.

Results

Reports on the use of a stent in dyssynergia are available.[23,24] A large multicentre study from North America[25] reported 153 cases of urodynamically diagnosed external sphincter dyssynergia in men with spinal cord injuries, 44 of whom (28.8%) had undergone at least one previous sphincterotomy. A 3 cm stent was used in all patients; 10 stents were removed following migration after implantation. Significant reductions in residual urine and voiding pressures occurred, with total bladder emptying and reduced voiding pressures being achieved in most patients. The stent became completely covered with urothelium within 3 months, but catheterization and endoscopy through the stent were still possible. Some patients developed bladder neck obstruction following stenting, which was resolved with a bladder neck incision. The use of this stent in conjunction with an artificial urinary sphincter appears to be limited.[26] In a direct comparison between sphincterotomy and stent insertion in 46 men with an injured spinal cord, 26 of whom elected to receive the stent, no difference was found in the degree of obstruction, voiding pressures or volume of residual urine on follow-up ranging from 6 to 20 months.[27] Complete urothelial covering was seen at 6 months. The authors concluded that stenting was as effective as sphincterotomy and was technically easier, cheaper and carried less morbidity.

Ten patients have been treated with a Memokath (Angiomed, Karlsruhe, Germany), a second-generation urethral stent manufactured from nitinol: complete bladder emptying was achieved in all patients. This stent is temporary and does not become covered with epithelium; long versions (7 cm) are available that will hold open both distal sphincter and bladder neck. Such stents need replacing periodically, but have the advantage that, in young patients, they can be removed to allow electroejaculation.[28]

Metal stents in prostatic disease

Benign prostatic hyperplasia (BPH) has a reported prevalence of 40% during the fifth decade of life, rising to 80% during the eighth decade.[29,30] It has been suggested that the chance of a 40-year-old man having a prostatectomy during his lifetime is 29%.[31–2] TURP is the traditional therapy of choice for symptomatic BPH, and remains the therapeutic modality with which all other therapies should be compared. It is a highly successful treatment, bringing about a 75–90% improvement in symptoms at 5 years.[33,34] Reoperation rates and mortality are associated with surgery.[35] Initially, stents were used for the treatment of outflow obstruction in those patients deemed unfit or unsuitable for surgery. Although many other less invasive modalities for treating prostate outflow obstruction are now available, including pharmacotherapy, thermotherapy, cryotherapy and high-frequency ultrasound, only stents relieve outflow obstruction to the same degree as surgery. Both temporary and permanent stents are available.

Temporary stents

In 1980, Fabian[36] first described the use of an indwelling urethral device to replace a permanent urethral catheter for the treatment of prostatic outflow obstruction. This device consists of a closely coiled spiral of stainless steel, narrowed at its inner end to allow introduction into the urethra. It has a single wire at its outer end, terminating at a smaller spiral and acting as a tail, to facilitate the adjustment of the position of the stent and to permit its easy removal (Fig. 8.20 and Fig. 8.21). The stent will become encrusted if left *in situ* for too long, and will not become epithelialized, in common with other temporary stents; cystocopy cannot be performed while the stent is in position. However, the stent, which is available in varying lengths, is a satisfactory temporary measure. Various modifications have been reported and results have been encouraging, although the technique of introduction has sometimes proved difficult. One modification has been developed by a Danish company (Engineers and Doctors). This stent, which is marketed as the Prostakath (Fig. 8.22), is gold-plated to reduce the rate of encrustation; nevertheless, encrustation will still occur if the stent is left *in situ* for too long. Other complications are haematuria, incontinence and urinary tract infection. A success rate of just over 50% can be expected, failure of the stent tending to occur in those with chronic retention who have a poorly functioning detrusor and who cannot generate sufficient intravesical pressure to overcome the resistance of the stent.[37]

In 1989 and 1990, Nissenkorn[38,39] described a urethral stent that consisted of a short double-Malecot 16 Fr polyurethane catheter (Fig. 8.23). The catheter lies within the prostatic urethra, with the inner Malecot at the bladder neck and the outer end of the catheter with its retaining device lying just distal to the verumontanum. The catheter is supplied in lengths of 45, 55 and 60 mm, and can be inserted under cystoscopic or transrectal ultrasound (TRUS) control. A small nylon suture can be threaded through the distal end of the stent and out through

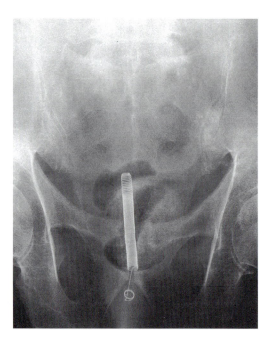

Figure 8.20
Plain film of the pelvis with a Prostakath in position.

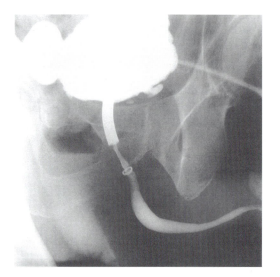

Figure 8.21
Suprapubic descending urethrogram with a Prostakath in position. The posterior urethra has an adequate calibre.

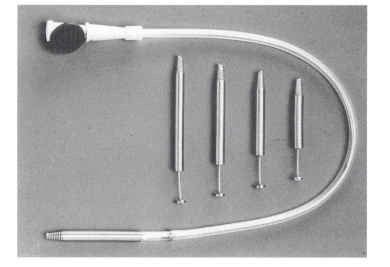

Figure 8.22
The Prostakath and its delivery device.

Figure 8.23
The Nissenkorn stent.

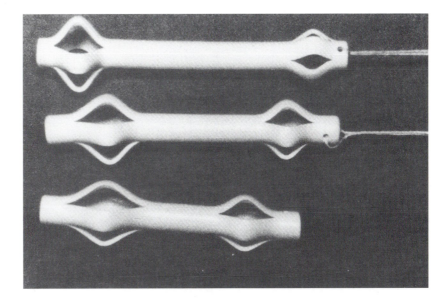

the external meatus; traction on the suture enables the stent to be removed. The stent is marketed by Angiomed (Karlsruhe, Germany) and can be left in situ for up to 18 weeks without any complications.

The use of a new biodegradable spiral stent in patients after laser ablation of the prostate has been reported recently.[40] The stent is manufactured from polyglycolic acid fibre formed into a spiral configuration similar in appearance to the Fabian stent described previously. The material degrades to glycolic acid by hydrolysis, the degradation time depending on the degree of polymerization and the internal arrangement of the material components at the site of implantation, and on the shape of the implant. Use of this stent has been reported in 22 patients treated with laser prostatectomy for BPH: it minimized voiding difficulties in the first few weeks of treatment. The development of biodegradable stents offers a means of temporarily relieving obstruction following laser prostatectomy, microwave treatment and cryotherapy. Such stents represent an exciting and valuable addition to the treatment options in obstruction of the prostatic urethra and potentially in other sites of the urinary tract.

Permanent stents

Two types of stent are available, one of which (the Urolume stent) is described above. The other type, exemplified by the Memotherm™ stent, is made of nickel–titanium alloy, using shape-metal technology: when the stent is cooled it is compressible, but when warmed to body temperature it expands to a flexible 42 Fr cylinder (Fig. 8.24). It is a variation of the vascular Strecker stent and is made from a single knitted wire; it can easily be removed by unravelling the wire.[41] The stent comes mounted on a 7 Fr catheter, and a simple gun-like deployment device (Fig. 8.25) allows its accurate placement (Fig. 8.26).

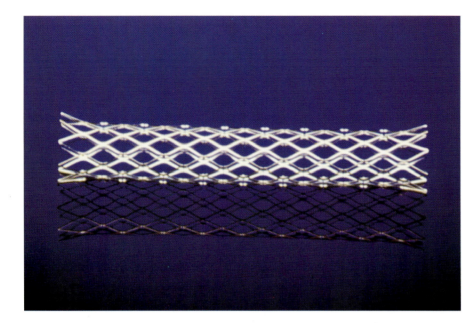

Figure 8.24
The nitinol Memotherm stent in its compressed form when cooled and in its decompressed form when warmed.

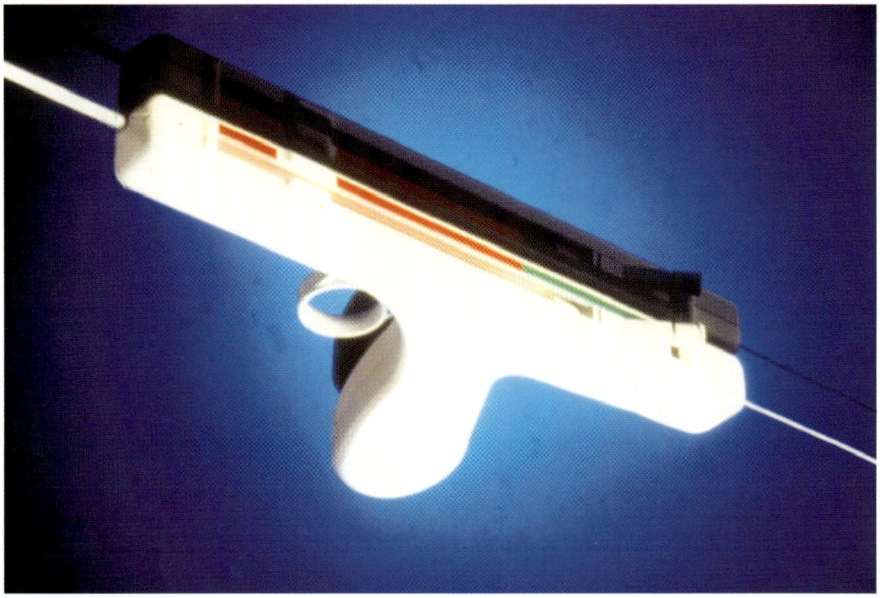

Figure 8.25
The Memotherm deployment device.

Indications for stent insertion

Originally, stents were used only in patients considered unfit for general anaesthesia. Early results of a multicentre randomized trial comparing the Urolume stent with TURP in patients fit for either procedure have shown that there is no significant difference in the postoperative symptoms, flow rates or re-treatment rates between the two groups.[42] The stent could therefore be considered as appropriate treatment in all patients with urodynamically significant BPH.

Figure 8.26
End-on view of a partially deployed Urolume Wallstent

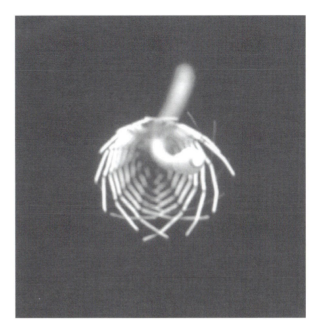

Pre-insertion imaging

Transrectal ultrasonography (TRUS) will give important information on prostate volume, the length of the posterior urethra and the relationship of the bladder neck to the bladder base. The presence of malignancy can be excluded by TRUS-guided biopsy. Urodynamic confirmation of the degree of outflow obstruction is also required.[43]

Urolume stent insertion for treatment of prostatic disease

Initially, stents were inserted under TRUS control (Fig. 8.27) but, because of the problem of inaccurate placement of the bladder end of the stent (Fig. 8.28), insertion under direct vision is preferred. The stent is preloaded on a specially designed insertion device. The length of the posterior urethra is measured endoscopically using a calibrated ureteric catheter and the appropriate stent size is introduced into the prostatic urethra under direct vision using a 0° telescope, as in the deployment of the stent in cases of urethral strictures. As before, stents with an unconstrained diameter of 14 mm (42 Fr) are used.

A stent 0.5 cm shorter than the distance from the bladder neck to the verumontanum should be selected. The delivery device is introduced into the prostatic urethra under direct vision and, when this is in position at the bladder neck, the first safety catch, which prevents premature opening of the stent, is released. Once the covering sheath of the stent has been pulled back as far as the second safety catch, the position of the stent is checked by moving the telescope along the full length of the stent, which then can be released. The verumontanum should be observed through the slots in the outer covering of the sheath. The relationship of the stent to the bladder neck, both anteriorly and posteriorly, is also checked (Fig. 8.29).

(a)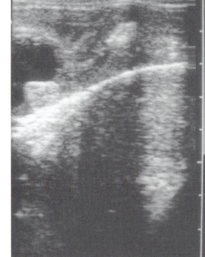
(b)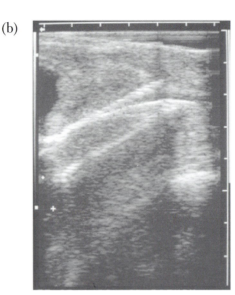

Figure 8.27
(a) Linear array TRUS image showing a partially deployed Urolume Wallstent lying just above the bladder neck. (b) Linear array TRUS image showing complete deployment of the stent within the posterior urethra.

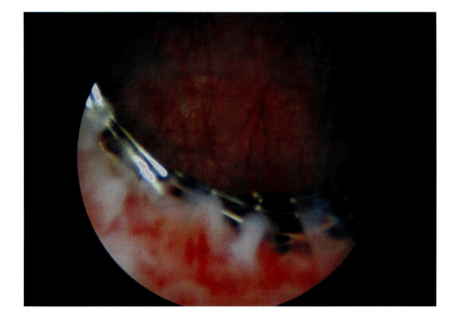

Figure 8.28
Endoscopic view of a misplaced stent. Free wires can be seen extending into the bladder. This will result in encrustation.

Complications of stent insertion in prostatic disease

Haematuria

Haematuria can occasionally cause clot retention immediately after stent insertion. Patients with this complication should be treated with a suprapubic catheter, which should be removed once the haematuria resolves. No urethral catheter should be passed for at least 1 month following stent insertion as this will risk displacement of, or damage to, the stent.

Retention

This is likely to occur in patients who develop postoperative clot retention, those who already have chronic retention of urine and those who have unstented apical

Figure 8.29
Endoscopic view of a Wallstent inserted under ultrasound control. Although there is good urothelial coating of the stent, free wires extend into the bladder. Eventually, encrustation will occur.

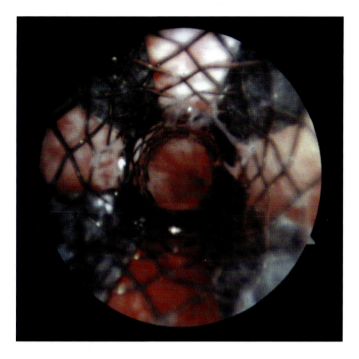

prostatic tissue. The first two groups should be treated with suprapubic catheterization. TRUS will identify uncovered apical tissue and a second overlapping stent can be inserted to relieve that source of obstruction.

Incontinence
Incontinence will occur if the stent is placed over the distal sphincter; care in placing the stent initially will guard against this. In patients with detrusor instability, the mechanical irritation of the stent may aggravate the condition, leading to incontinence; this may be relieved by the use of oxybutynin.

Ejaculatory function
A surprising feature of the Urolume prostatic stent is the low incidence of retrograde ejaculation – a common symptom in patients undergoing TURP. Antegrade ejaculation in fit, sexually active patients can be expected in 80% of patients in whom Urolume stents are inserted.

Intrastent hyperplasia
Following stent insertion, a variable amount of epithelial hyperplasia occurs, but settles spontaneously between 6 and 12 months later (Fig. 8.30 and Fig. 8.31). When the hyperplasia is mild, no problems will be encountered; occasionally, however, it is severe and causes significant outflow obstruction. This is more common in the prostate than in the treatment of urethral strictures.

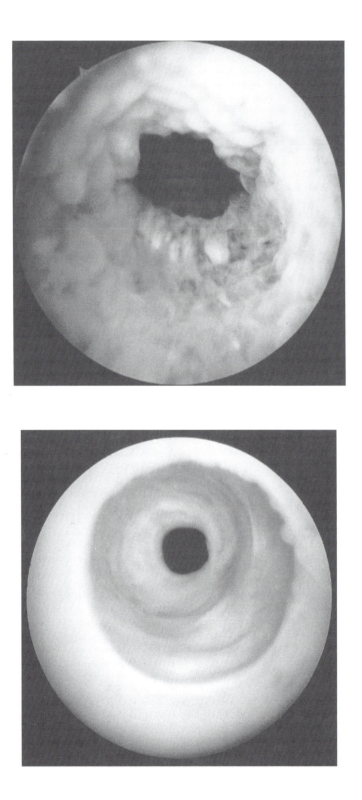

Figure 8.30
Endoscopic view of the Urolume stent being deployed within the posterior urethra.

Figure 8.31
Endoscopic view of a Urolume stent in the posterior urethra 3 months after insertion, showing hyperplasia.

Contraindications

Prostatic stents should not be used in patients who have very large prostates and superior extension of the central part of the gland – the so-called middle lobe: in such cases the stent tends to move to the anterior half of the urethra, resulting in split urethra. Although most of the stent becomes covered with endothelium, wires crossing between large lateral lobes may not become covered completely, with resultant encrustation.

Stent removal

The stent is easily removed if it is not covered with urothelium, using a specifically designed grasping device. Alternatively, a guidewire can be passed through the wall of the stent into the bladder and the stent pushed into the bladder; the free end of the guidewire can then be grasped and the wire, stent and endoscopic sheath all removed together.[44] Stents covered with urothelium within the prostate can be removed using rigid crocodile forceps within a nephroscope sheath; the stent can be freed from the surrounding prostatic tissue and removed intact.[45]

Postinsertion imaging

Transrectal ultrasound
Temporary stents have a closely woven mesh that attenuates the ultrasound beam to such an extent that it is not possible to image the intrastent lumen or the relationship of the stent to the bladder neck (Fig. 8.32), which is best done by urethrography. The position of permanent stents can be clearly defined by TRUS. For accurate scanning, the bladder needs to be part full (Fig. 8.33); this will enable very accurate depiction of the relationship of the stent to the bladder neck. The position of the distal end of the stent and its relationship to the distal sphincter and apical prostatic tissue can be assessed precisely (Fig. 8.34). Postoperative incontinence may be due to pre-existing bladder instability, instability as a result of instrumentation, or compromise of distal sphincter function because the stent is partly or wholly covering it; TRUS will help to differentiate between poor positioning and a functional abnormality. As mentioned earlier, in the first few months following insertion, permanent stents invoke a hyperplastic covering, the extent and uniformity of which can be

Figure 8.32
Transrectal ultrasound of a temporary stent. The close knit of the stent attenuates the ultrasound beam to such an extent that accurate imaging is not possible.

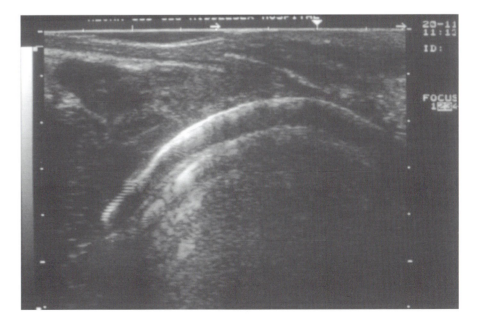

(a)

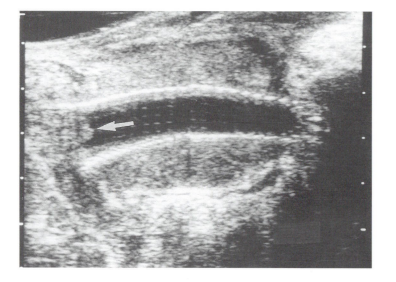

(b)

Figure 8.33
(a) TRUS image of a Urolume stent in a good position. Its relationship to the bladder neck cannot be assessed with the bladder empty. There is herniation of bladder mucosa into the stent (arrow). (b) Linear array TRUS image of a Urolume stent 4 years after insertion, showing smooth urothelial covering. The relationship of the stent to the bladder neck (top left) and to the distal sphincter (bottom right) is good.

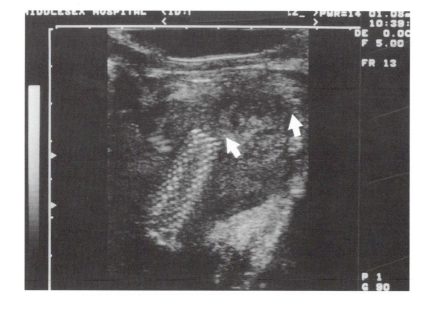

Figure 8.34
Linear array TRUS image of a Prostakath stent.

assessed by TRUS. Usually, the stent is covered by urothelium 1–2 mm thick, leaving an adequate intrastent lumen, but occasional focal areas of overgrowth are seen. Colour-Doppler imaging (CDI) in the transverse axial or forward-looking sagittal planes can be used to assess the vascularity of the neo-urothelium (Fig. 8.35).

Misplacement of the stent at the bladder neck, resulting in free wires not in contact with urothelium, may lead to encrustation; TRUS will demonstrate such free wires and show whether small stones are forming on them. Perineal pain following stent insertion may be due to the development of prostatic inflammatory disease, prostatic abscess or blockage of the prostatic or ejaculatory ducts; TRUS will differentiate between these entities and point the clinician to the appropriate therapeutic course. Prolonged haematuria following stent insertion may be caused by prominent vessels supplying the urothelial covering; TRUS, combined with CDI, will demonstrate such vessels.

Figure 8.35
(a) Linear array colour-Doppler TRUS image of a Urolume stent 3 months after insertion in a patient with haematuria. Prominent intrastent vessels can be seen. (b) Endoscopic view of the same patient, showing the bleeding vessels.

(a)

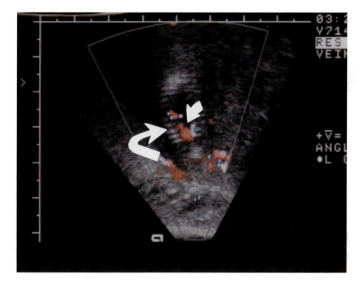

(b)

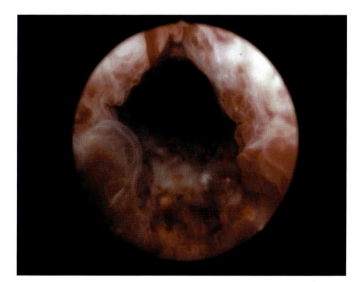

Urethrography

In the first few weeks following insertion, hyperplasia will cause irregular intrastent narrowing; however, when the urothelial covering is complete, the intrastent lumen becomes smooth. The relationship of the distal end of the stent to the distal sphincter can be assessed on ascending studies, but is best demonstrated on descending studies during interruption of micturition.

Long-term results with the Urolume prostatic stent

The authors have inserted over 150 stents in patients with BPH. Review of the first 54 patients (the majority of whom presented with urinary retention) at a mean follow-up of 12 months showed that 44 were passing urine satisfactorily and were satisfied with their treatment. The stents became fully covered with urothelium between 6 and 9 months following insertion. Six stents had to be removed because of severe detrusor instability or persisting incontinence. In 44 patients reported by Bahoria,[46] 4 stents had to be removed as a result of stent migration or displacement. In the remaining patients good relief of obstruction was obtained; full epithelial covering of the stent was seen in all but 3 patients at 6 months and in one further patient at 12 months.

Stents in prostatic disease: conclusions

Permanent prostatic stents, such as the Urolume, give better relief of obstruction than drug treatment, balloon dilatation, hyperthermia or thermotherapy. Compared with temporary stents, they have the great advantage of becoming covered with urothelium, which will resist encrustation and infection; thus, they do not require regular replacement and can be regarded as a permanent means of relief of obstruction. Longer follow-up is required to define more accurately the indications for stents in the treatment of BPH. At present, it seems reasonable to offer permanent prostatic stents to fit, elderly patients as an alternative to prostatic surgery.

References

1   Siwart U, Puel J, Mirkovitch V, Joffre F, Kappenberger L. Intravascular stents to prevent occlusion and restenosis after transluminal angioplasty. *N Engl J Med* 1987; **316**: 701.
2   Milroy EJG, Chapple CR, Cooper JE *et al*. A new treatment for urethral strictures. *Lancet* 1988; **1**: 1424.
3   Hunter J. Treatise on venereal disease. In: Palmer JF (ed) *The works of John Hunter FRS*, vol. 2, London: Longman, Rees, Orme, Brown, Green and Longman, 1935.
4   Attwater HL. The history of urethral stricture. *Br J Urol* 1943; **15**: 39–51.
5   Otis FN. Remarks on strictures of the urethra of extreme caliber, with cases and a description of new instruments for their treatment. *NY State Med J* 1872; **15**: 152.
6   Petersen NE. Traumatic posterior urethral avulsion. *Monogr Urol* 1986: 61–82.
7   Konnak JW, Kogan BA. Otis internal urethrotomy in the treatment of urethral stricture disease. *J Urol* 1980; **121**: 356.
8   Lapides J, Diokno, AL, Siber SJ. Clean intermittent self catheterisation in the treatment of urinary tract disease. *J Urol* 1972; **107**: 458.
9   Harrison NW, De Souza JV. Prostatic stenting for outflow obstruction. *Br J Urol* 1990; **65**: 192–196.
10 Sarramon JP, Joffre F, Rischmann P, Rousseau H, Eldin A, Wallsten H. The Wallstent endoprothesis for recurrent urethral strictures. *Ann Urol (Paris)* 1989; **38**: 383–387.
11 Bosnjakovic P, Ilic M, Ivkovic T *et al*. Flexible Tantalum stents: effects in the stenotic canine urethra. *Cardiovasc Intervent Radiol* 1994; **17**: 280–284.

12 Latal D, Moraz J, Zerhau P, Susani M, Marberger M. Nitinol urethral stents: long term results in dogs. *Urol Res* 1994; **22**: 295–300.

13 Yachia D, Bayar M. Temporarily implanted coil stent for the treatment of recurrent urethral strictures: a preliminary report. *J Urol* 1991; **146**: 1001–1004.

14 Yachia D, Aridogan IA, Erlich N. Long term follow up urethral strictures treated with a removable urethral stent of the Urocoil system. *J Urol* 1995; **153**: 373A.

15 Kempainen E, Talja M, Riihela M, Pohjonen T, Tormala P, Alfthan O. Bioresorbable urethral stent: an experimental study. *Urol Res* 1993; **21**: 235–238.

16 Donald JJ, Rickards D, Milroy EJG. Stricture disease: radiology of urethral stents. *Radiology* 1991; **180**: 447–450.

17 Parikh AM, Milroy EJG. Precautions and complications in the use of the Urolome Wallstent. *Eur Urol* 1995; **563**: 1–13.

18 Milroy EJG, Chapple CR, Cooper JE *et al.* A new treatment for urethral strictures. *Lancet* 1988; **1**: 1424–1427.

19 Ashken MH, Coulange C, Milroy EJG, Sarramon JP. European experience with the urethral Wallstent for urethral strictures. *Eur Urol* 1991; **19**: 181.

20 Badlani G, Press SM, Oesterling JE, DeFalco K. Urolume endothelial prosthesis for the treatment of urethral stricture disease: long term results of the North American multi-center Urolume trial. *Urology* 1995; **45**: 846.

21 Milroy E, Allen A. Long-term results of Urolume urethral stent for recurrent urethral strictures. *J Urol* 1995; **155**: 156–161.

22 Breda G, Xausa D, Pupo P *et al.* Urolume in ureteral stenosis: Italian club of minimally invasive urology experience. *J Endourol* 1994; **8**: 305–309.

23 Shaw PJR, Milroy EJG, Timoney AG, El Din A, Mitchell N. Permanent external striated sphincter stents in patients with spinal injuries. *Br J Urol* 1990; **66**: 297–302.

24 McInerney PD, Vanner TF, Harris SAB, Stephenson TP. Permanent urethral stents for detrusor sphincter dyssynergia. *Br J Urol* 1991; **67**: 291–294.

25 Chancellor MB, Rivas DA, Linsenneyer T *et al.* Multi-centre trial in North America of the Urolume urinary sphincter. *J Urol* 1994; **152**: 924–930.

26 Chancellor MB, Karusick S, Erhard MJ *et al.* Placement of a wire mesh prosthesis in the external urinary sphincter of men with spinal cord injuries. *Radiology* 1993; **187**: 551–555.

27 Rivas DA, Chancellor MB, Bagley D. Prospective comparison of external sphincter prosthesis placement and external sphincterotomy in men with spinal cord injury. *J Endourol* 1994; **8**: 89–93.

28 Soni BM, Vaidyanatham S, Krishnan KR. Use of Memokath, a second generation urethral stent for relief of urinary retention in male spinal cord injured patients. *Paraplegia* 1994; **32**: 480–488.

29 Moore RA. The morphology of small prostatic carcinoma. *J Urol* 1935; **33**: 224–234.

30 Franks LM. Benign nodular hyperplasia of the prostate: a review. *Ann R Coll Surg Engl* 1954; **14**: 92–106.

31 Glynn RJ, Champion EW, Bouchard GR, Silbert JE. The development of benign prostatic hyperplasia among volunteers in the normative aging study. *Am J Epidemiol* 1985; **121**: 78–82.

32 Mebust WK. Surgical management of benign prostatic obstruction. *Urology* 1988; **32**(Suppl.): 12–15.

33 Bruskewitz RC, Larsen EH, Madsen PO. Three year follow-up of urinary symptoms after transurethral resection of the prostate. *J Urol* 1986; **136**: 613–615.

34 Meyhoff HH. Transurethral versus transvesical prostatectomy: clinical urodynamic, renographic and economic aspects: a randomised study. *Scand J Urol Nephrol* 1987; **102**(Suppl.): 1–26.

35 Roos NP, Wennberg JE, Malenka DJ. Mortality and reoperation after open and transurethral resection of the prostate for benign prostatic hyperplasia. *N Engl J Med* 1989; **320**: 1120–1123.

36 Fabian KM. Der interprostatische 'patielle Katheter' (urologische Spirale). *Urologe* 1980; **19**: 236–238.

37 Harrison NW, De Souza JV. Prostatic stenting for outflow obstruction. *Br J Urol* 1990; **65**: 192–196.

38 Nissenkorn I. Experience with a new self-retaining urethral catheter in patients with chronic retention. *J Urol* 1989; **142**: 92–94.

39 Nissenkorn I, Richter S. A self-retaining intra-urethral device. *Br J Urol* 1990; **65**: 197–200.

40 Talja M, Tammela T, Petas A *et al.* Biodegradable self reinforced polyglycolic acid spiral stent in the prevention of postoperative urinary retention after visual laser ablation of the prostate — laser prostatectomy. *J Urol* 1995; **154**: 2089–2092.

41 Chapple CR, Milroy EJG, Rickards D. Use of endourological stents in the management of benign prostatic hyperplasia. *Semin Intervent Radiol* 1991; **8**: 283.

42 Chapple CR, Rossario DJ, Wasserfallen M, Woo HH, Nordling J, Milroy EJG. A randomised study of the Urolume stent and prostatic surgery. *J Urol* 1995; **153**: 436A.

43 Rickards D. Recent advances in ultrasound. In: Kirby R S, Hendry W F (eds). *Recent advances in urology and andrology*, vol. 5 London: Churchill Livingstone, 1994: 25–35.

44 Parikh AM, Milroy EJG. A new technique for removal of the Urolume prostate stent. *Br J Urol* 1993; **71**: 620–626.

45 Anjum MI, Palmer JH. A technique for removal of the Urolume endourethral prosthesis. *Br J Urol* 1995; **76**: 655–656.

46 Bahoria S, Agarwal SA, White R, Zafar F, Williams G. Experience with the second generation Urolume prostatic stent. *Br J Urol* 1995; **75**: 325–327.

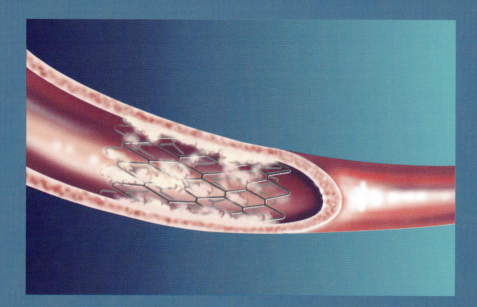

Chapter 9
Biological effects of metallic stents

H.H. Schild and H. Strunk

Introduction

Stents are designed to keep dilated or recanalized lumina open, when dilatation or recanalization alone do not achieve the desired result. The main areas for stent implantation in interventional radiology are the vascular system and the biliary tree. Less frequently, stents are deployed into other regions, such as the tracheobronchial system, genitourinary tract and gastrointestinal tract. This chapter focuses on the biological effects of metallic stents in the areas of most interest to the interventional radiologist, with emphasis on the vascular system.*

Vascular stents

Vascular stents are more or less embedded into the vessel wall at the time of deployment. The endovascular manipulations involved inevitably affect the internal vessel lining: endothelium is damaged, or the vessel is completely denuded from this covering layer. In an attempt to repair the damage, a new intima develops, which becomes covered by a new endothelium. Finally, the stent is also covered by this new lining and is no more in contact with the flowing blood. The processes involved are rather complex. They may be disturbed at various levels, which can be the cause of clinical problems. In the extreme, such disturbances may result in stent occlusion, which may be due to either thrombus formation or intimal hyperplasia. While thrombotic occlusions are usually seen in the early course, problems resulting from intimal hyperplasia are typically observed months after stent implantation. In the following, such stent occlusions are used as models to explain and discuss the biological effects of metallic stents in the vascular system.

Thrombotic stent occlusion

Endovascular manipulations during stent placement cause unavoidable endothelial damage. This exposes subendothelial tissues, which are thrombogenic, to the bloodstream. The result is activation of the coagulation system and concurrent thrombus formation.[1,2] However, it is not only the

---

*Much of the present knowledge about the biological effects of metallic stents comes from work by Julio Palmaz, to whom the authors want to give special credit.

exposure of subendothelial tissues that activates the coagulation system: the stents themselves also are thrombogenic.[3]

Stent thrombogenicity is influenced by various factors:[4] surface texture; electrical surface charge; free surface energy; and stent expansion.

The surface texture of a stent[5] directly influences thrombogenicity: the smoother the stent surface the less thrombogenic it is, and vice versa.

Electrical surface charge is a factor with which physicians are usually not so familiar. Intravascular surfaces (endothelium) usually have an electronegative charge, as is also true for cells and proteins in the blood. Because of their similar charge, repelling forces exist that keep blood cells and proteins away from the endothelium to a certain degree.[6] Most metals or alloys used for stents (or intravascular devices in general) have a positive surface charge. When exposed to blood, they do not repel but attract negatively charged proteins and cells. Within minutes, this leads to a thin film at the stent surface, consisting mainly of proteins, especially of fibrinogen. This film serves to neutralize the electrical charges, i.e. 'passivates' the stent surface.[7]

The plasma proteins in this film possess reactive groups that bind platelets, with the latter promoting further protein deposition.[8] Larger blood cells also attach to this layer, depending on local flow patterns and shear stress (see below). Unlike most other metals, tantalum, which is used, for example, in the construction of the Strecker stent (Boston Scientific Inc., Watertown, MA, USA), has an electronegative surface charge after thorough cleaning during the manufacturing process.[9,10] This, however, is of no practical advantage, as the material becomes electropositive within a few hours when exposed to electrolyte solutions, such as blood.[5] Under normal flow conditions, the thrombus developing at the stent surface is not very extensive and consists mainly of platelet aggregates. It is not very stable, and easily reversible.[11]

The protein film at the stent surface not only serves to reduce its thrombogenicity, it is also necessary for stent endothelialization to occur, as endothelial cells cannot grow on the naked metal surface. When the stent is finally covered by endothelium, it is completely isolated from the bloodstream and consequently no longer thrombogenic.

Free surface energy is another physicochemical property influencing the biological behaviour of stents. It is related to unsatisfied intermolecular bonds at the material surface, and largely determines how well a fluid is spread over the material (its 'wettability'). It may be measured as critical surface tension (in dyn/cm; 1 dyn = 10 μN). If this is above 20–30 dyn/cm – as is the case for most metals – the material is thrombogenic.[12] Interestingly enough, the fibrinogen film developing on the stent after deployment into the bloodstream changes the critical surface tension of the metal surface to within the thromboresistant range.

The degree of expansion of a stent also influences its thrombogenicity, albeit indirectly. With ideal expansion, the metal struts of a stent should be pressed into the vessel wall. Next to the struts, depressions in the vascular wall result. These will fill with thrombus, covering the corresponding stent surface. In between the struts, tissue mounds protrude towards the vessel lumen. If these retain their endothelium, this can be the origin of multicentre re-endothelialization.

It becomes obvious that as much normal endothelium as possible should remain in the stented segment. In other words, in a stented vessel the surface area covered by metal should be kept minimal, while the free luminal surface should be maximized. This ratio between metal covered and free surface area is called the 'aspect ratio' and should also be minimized.[13] Stents with the least metal also show less stenosis and intimal hyperplasia during follow-up, as is discussed later.[14] Unfortunately, the aspect ratio becomes less favourable with decreasing stent size; this holds true for stents designed for small-diameter vessels, as well as for incompletely expanded stents.[15–17] If stent expansion is insufficient, more of the stent framework will be facing the bloodstream. This causes more extensive thrombus deposition, which can form a continuous layer covering all of the stented vessel segment. In this case re-endothelialization can only occur from the endothelium in the unaffected vessel next to the stent or from unaffected sidebranches. As this process takes longer than multicentre endothelialization, chances for thrombus formation and intimal hyperplasia (see page 178) and, consequently, stent failure, are increased.

Metallic stents and haemodynamics

Beside the endoluminal damage caused by stent implantation, and the stent properties mentioned, other factors influence/contribute to thrombus formation during and after stent implantation. *Haemodynamic factors* play an important role: blood flow, flow velocity and shear stress directly or indirectly influence events.[11]

With laminar flow, flow velocity increases towards the centre of a vessel. This corresponds to the parabolic flow profile over a vascular cross-section. Between the endothelium and the fluid layer next to it, as well as between contiguous fluid layers, shear stresses of varying degree result. All of this contributes to the so-called axial accumulation of blood cells: not unlike ships on a river, blood cells are preferably located towards the vessel centre under normal flow conditions.[18]

When flow velocity decreases, or when laminar flow becomes turbulent, axial accumulation of blood cells is less pronounced and finally disappears. Platelets, erythrocytes and others move closer to the endothelium. If this is damaged, contact with the thrombogenic subendothelial tissues is intensified. Increased platelet and coagulation activation are the consequences.[19] In addition, because of slower flow and localized areas of turbulence, activated coagulation factors are not washed out from the site of activation as fast as normal. The decreased flow and resulting diminished shear stress, as well as localized areas of turbulence, lead to a more stable thrombus that contains more fibrin and red blood cells. The amount of this thrombus increases with decreasing shear stress.[11]

Under certain circumstances, this increase in thrombus can be considered an adaptive response. This has been demonstrated experimentally when stent diameters significantly exceeded the dimension of the target vessel.[16] In the stented area, flow was slowed down with a resulting rise in thrombus formation. This in turn led to luminal narrowing and consecutive increase in flow velocity to a level above a thrombogenic threshold. In general, areas with abnormal flow conditions or reduced flow are more prone to develop extensive thrombus, and thus have a greater risk for thrombotic stent occlusion.

Stent occlusion by intimal hyperplasia

Formation of a neointima can be considered a normal repair process, triggered by damage to the vessel wall.[20–2] The endovascular manipulations during stent implantation inevitably damage the endothelium. Resulting exposure of the subendothelial tissues, as well as the stent itself, initiate and promote some thrombus formation, as mentioned before. Initially, this thrombus has a tendency to especially cover zones of turbulence, and irregularities.[23] Platelets that adhere to the injured site release the 'platelet derived growth factor' (PDGF). This is a potent vascular smooth muscle cell chemoattractant and mitogen.[24,25] It causes smooth muscle cells from the media to proliferate, after which they migrate through natural openings in the internal elastic lamina towards the luminal side of the vessel wall. Subsequently, they proliferate to form a neointima. In a rat model, the proliferation maximum in the media was seen after 24 hours, while in the intima it was observed after 96 hours.[26,27] As smooth muscle cell proliferation continues well beyond the interval of platelet deposition, other mechanisms than PDGF must also be involved. Experimental evidence suggests other sources of PDGF, e.g. the media muscle cells themselves, endothelial cells, and also macrophages. The latter, however, seem to play no major role. The mechanism of PDGF release from these cells is unclear. A feedback system under the control of the circumferential wall stress is discussed.[28] In addition, other factors, e.g. fibroblast growth factor, contribute to the events.[29]

Whatever the underlying mechanism, the resulting neointima is characterized by an increased permeability. This allows for easier and longer diffusion of growth factors, at least while the endothelial cover is still deficient. At the time of neointimal proliferation re-endothelialization also occurs.[30] The new endothelium originates from intact endothelium outside the stented vessel segment, including sidebranches, and from endothelium located on the tissue mounds protruding between the stent struts.[31] In the case of extensive thrombus formation, re-endothelialization can only start from endothelium in the unaffected vessels next to the stent.

Notwithstanding their origin, the endothelial cells spreading over the damaged vessel surface initially consist of a mixture of polygonal and elongated cells, without preferred orientation.[32] During the next weeks, the endothelial cells mature; they become flat and elongated, and finally are orientated in the direction of the blood flow. To a certain extent, the integrity and function of this endothelium are influenced by local flow conditions. With inadequate or no flow, the endothelial cells will be deformed and have a rougher surface.[33] This is more prone to platelet adherence and may in turn explain the more frequent thrombotic problems in stents deployed under reduced flow conditions.[34] With complete endothelialization,[35] growth factors originating from the luminal side, such as those from platelets and macrophages, can no more stimulate the vascular smooth muscle cells.

The time necessary for complete endothelialization varies, depending for example on the stent dimensions. Stents with struts of 0.1 mm diameter are completely covered in 3–4 weeks. If struts have a diameter of 0.45 mm, only 30% of the surface is covered by endothelium in about a month.[36–8] Eventually, all of the thrombotic material resulting from stent deployment is replaced by the fibromuscular cells and intercellular matrix of the neointima. A damaged elastic lamina will not be restored.[39]

The neointimal layer plateaus in thickness several months after stenting in most animal studies. Its maximum thickness has been observed between 2 and 6 months after stent placement.[40–3]

Later, the thickness of the neointima may decrease. This has been observed in some experimental as well as clinical studies, and may be accompanied by an increase in vessel lumen. The underlying processes are not completely understood. However, in specimens obtained years after stent implantation, the neointima contained mostly collagen and some fibrocytes. This composition resembles that of scar tissue elsewhere in the body. It may be speculated that transformation into this 'scar tissue' causes the decrease in neointimal thickness, comparable to the shrinkage of other scars with time.

For reasons as yet incompletely understood, neointima formation may be excessive, leading to stent stenosis and finally occlusion. Interestingly enough, this restenosis frequently develops at the side of the former native vessel narrowing. It can be speculated that in these cases stent implantation did not resolve the underlying (haemodynamic?) problem that was causing the initial lesion.

More obvious reasons for excessive intimal hyperplasia are abrupt changes in diameter or direction between the stented and unstented vessel segments. This can be regarded as an attempt to smooth out transitions. Modelling the wall by means of neointimal hyperplasia results in a more uniform vessel diameter with less abrupt changes in flow direction.[18]

Prevention and treatment of neointimal hyperplasia

Neointimal hyperplasia is a normal consequence of a repair process triggered by damage to the vessel wall. Excessive neointimal hyperplasia, however, is one of the main reasons for restenosis (and reocclusion) after successful balloon angioplasty as well as after stent implantation. Initially it was speculated that rigid stents like the Palmaz™ stent (Johnson & Johnson, Warren, NJ, USA) lead to less intimal hyperplasia, and thus to a lower frequency of restenosis.[44,45] However, it is still open to debate whether rigid or flexible stents cause more intimal hyperplasia.[46]

Various attempts to reduce or influence intimal hyperplasia have been made experimentally as well as clinically. All of them focus on known steps involved in neointima formation. Proliferation of the involved media muscle cells at least initially depends on platelet adherence and release of various growth factors, especially PDGF. Prevention or reduction of platelet aggregation reduces this stimulus, perhaps limiting the neointimal proliferation.[13,15] Consequently, patients should receive drugs to reduce platelet aggregation and/or platelet function before, during and after stent placement.[47,48]

Experimentally, it has been shown that low-level radioactivity can completely inhibit neointimal proliferation. As proliferation occurs over several weeks, the study concluded that radiation should extend over a comparable time.[49,50] In clinical studies, a decrease in intimal hyperplasia after single endoluminal treatments with local doses of about 12 Gy has been reported.[51] Antibodies against PDGF have also been produced and tested with some effect.[27] Also it has been demonstrated that metal ions, such as copper, leaking from the stent surface, may cause more extensive intimal hyperplasia; these, perhaps, act as cofactors in enzymatic processses.[52] Consequently, stent materials should be stable in order to minimize such effects.

When excessive intimal hyperplasia has occurred and is the cause of stenosis within a stent, this may be treated with atherectomy devices, removing as much as possible of the obstructing material. Frequently, however, balloon angioplasty alone leads to improvement. The underlying mechanism may be re-expansion of a compressed and narrowed stent, or compression of protruding hyperplastic intimal tissue.[53]

It has been demonstrated that about 85% of the improvement is due to tissue compression and extrusion through stent interstices, and about 15% is caused by stent expansion.[54] In addition, balloon-induced intimal remodelling characterized by focal intimal tearing and mild intramural haemorrhage may be observed.

Effects of metallic stents on the abluminal side of the vessel

All the processes and problems described preferentially involve the luminal stent side and are mainly based on interactions with the bloodstream. However, stents also cause effects on their abluminal side.[55] These effects are not restricted only to stent struts invading deeper layers of the vessel wall, as may be observed at the end of Wallstent™ endoprostheses (Schneider, Minneapolis, MN, USA):[56] a number of other effects may also be seen. The intima and the luminal half of the media are supplied by diffusion from the vessel lumen, the other layers via vasa vasorum. Usually, beyond a distance of 0.5 mm from the lumen, the arterial wall is vascularized. With regard to oxygenation, the middle zone of the media is the most critical. This situation may become aggravated after a stent implantation, for various reasons. The distance to the vessel lumen increases because of the neointima formation. Vasa vasorum may be compressed, and the oxygen demand of the vessel wall increases because of the proliferation and migration of smooth muscle cells. As an adaptive response, the number of vasa vasorum increases, leading to greater vascularity of stented arterial walls.[57–9]

Beneath the stent struts the tunica media may become thinned and apparently atrophic. In an experimental setting, media thickness in stented vessels averaged 100–150 μm whereas that in unstented vessels averaged 300–400 μm. Simple stretching with consecutive thinning of the vessel wall cannot in itself account for this difference.[60] Instead, the decrease in media thickness may be due to physical compression by the expanding stent, leading to medial thinning and necrosis. In addition, the media atrophies, as smooth muscle stretching by pulsatile flow (acting as a stimulant) is reduced beneath the relatively stiff stents.[61]

This stiffness of metallic stents generally influences the mechanical properties of the vessel at the implantation site. Vascular compliance is reduced after stent implantation.[60] This means that an increase in transmural pressure causes less increase in vessel diameter than normal.[62] In other words, the pulsatile diameter change in stented vessels becomes markedly reduced, and there is more loss of pulsatile energy at the stented segment compared with a normal vessel. Impedance to local flow is increased. This results in greater pressure wave reflections and pulsatile mechanical stress at the interface between stented and non-stented vessel segments. On a microscopic level, this leads to locally increased velocity gradients and areas of turbulence, with vibratory weakening of the arterial wall. This, in turn, causes greater local stress, leading to endothelial damage,[62] and pronounced neointima formation as the final consequence of the compliance mismatch. A similar mechanism has also been blamed for the high incidence of graft failures in small-diameter vascular prosthetic grafts.[63,64]

Metal stents and intrahepatic portosystemic shunts

The biological effects of metal stents used for creation of intrahepatic portosystemic shunts are in some regards quite similar to those in the vascular system.[65] Shortly after stent deployment there will be fresh thrombus adhering to the stent mesh. A few days later, the stented tracts will have an irregular luminal surface, with liver parenchyma protruding between stent struts and with a patchy layer of intimal cells.[66] After about three weeks, the stent wires are covered by a pseudointimal surface. This is composed of granulation tissue and a contiguous layer of endothelial cells. The extent of the pseudointima formation is variable, with the neointimal layer measuring 440–600 μm in thickness. After approximately three months, the neointima consists mainly of densely collagenized scar tissue.[67,68] When shunts become stenotic, hyperplastic pseudointima, measuring more than 5 mm in thickness, may be seen. In an animal model, stenoses were mainly caused by progressive proliferation of fibrous tissue.[69,70]

Biological effects of metallic stents: practical consequences

From the described reactions to metallic stent implantation some conclusions for everyday practice may be drawn:[18]

1 The material-dependent thrombogenicity of the stent should be kept at a minimum. It should not be increased by suboptimal handling, e.g. grasping it with a metal forceps and damaging the smooth surface which is a prerequisite for an uncomplicated proteinaceous cover and endothelialization.
2 All endovascular manipulations should be performed very carefully, to minimize endothelial trauma and the consecutive stimulus for thrombus formation.
3 Administration of platelet aggregation inhibitors should be started the day before stent implantation. The procedure should also be carried out under heparinization, which should also cover the first 24–36 hours after stent placement. This minimizes the amount of inevitable thrombus formation at the stented site and the risk of thrombotic stent occlusion. As the platelets stimulate proliferation by PDGFs, minimizing platelet accumulation may also have a direct effect on the amount of intimal hyperplasia.

Prevention/reduction of coagulation and thrombus formation is especially important when stents are used under impaired flow conditions or for recanalization:

1 Slow or reduced flow, as well as turbulence, promotes thrombus formation and its consequences.
2 Occluded vessels lack normal endothelium. After stent deployment there are no tissue mounds with normal endothelium protruding through the stent. Instead, the tissues exposed to the blood have a higher thrombogenicity as they lack normal endothelium.[71] The risk for thrombus formation is increased, and also exists over a longer time period, as the normal multicentre endothelialization is impossible, and re-endothelialization requires more time.
3 Stent dimensions should be appropriate. The stent should cover the area to be treated, but not deliberately extend to neighbouring healthy areas. This would only contribute to coagulation activation and neointimal hyperplasia.
4 The stent diameter should also be appropriate. About 1.2 times the vessel diameter is recommended, as this ensures satisfactory embedding of the struts into the vessel wall. With incomplete stent embedding, formation of fibrin and thrombus along the stent is increased. This in turn promotes (sub-) occlusive thrombus formation, and also intimal hyperplasia.[71]

   If the stent diameter is more than 20–30% greater than the vessel diameter, there is more damage to the vessel wall and vessel spasms are seen more frequently. The risk of thrombus formation and trauma-induced intimal hyperplasia is increased, and consequently so is the likelihood of restenosis.[72] Excessive expansion pressure of the stent may predispose to more pronounced neointimal hyperplasia; however, this is not generally accepted.[56]

5   Transition between stented and unstented segments should be smooth. Pronounced changes in calibre, as well as direction, should also be avoided. With abrupt changes in diameter or direction, intimal hyperplasia becomes more pronounced. This adaptive response may be beneficial under certain circumstances. However, it constitutes an unnecessary stimulus for proliferation, and development of vessel or stent stenosis.

6   With regard to anticoagulation after stent implantation, various facts have to be considered. Anticoagulation should be performed when stents are placed in critical vessels, in case of recanalization, or when implantation under impeded flow conditions is performed.[71] Anticoagulation should be given as long as there is a risk of thrombotic stent occlusion, i.e. as long as the stent is not completely insulated from the flowing blood by endothelialization. Most stents that are used intra-arterially will be covered by neointima in a matter of 4–6 weeks. To be on the safe side, platelet inhibitors should be given for at least 6 months, and coumarin administration should also extend over this time period.

7   At present, there are no recommendations for antibiotic prophylaxis under certain circumstances, e.g. tooth extractions. However, this should be considered on an individual basis.[18]

Biliary stents

Placement of metallic stents into the biliary tract has become an established form of therapy in certain forms of biliary obstruction. As in the vascular system, stent placement also leads to unavoidable injury to the biliary tree on a microscopic level. The epithelial damage initiates mucosal proliferations. These proliferations advance like tentacles through the spaces in between the stent struts. With time, these protrusions may coalesce, while the stent may become more embedded into the wall, i.e. into the superficial submucosal layer. With stent position in the submucosa, the mucosal thickening decreases, as has been shown in canine studies.[73]

Focal compression of tissue and reactive inflammatory processes resembling foreign body reactions in the wall may be observed histologically.[74]

Tracheobronchial stents

The events after stent implantation into the tracheobronchial system are to a certain degree modified by the situation before stenting. When a stent is deployed into an area that was treated in some way immediately before stent placement (e.g. laser therapy of an obstructing tumour), the situation differs from that when stents are placed on a normal mucosa.

When placed on more or less normal mucosa, the stent struts cause impressions that vary in extent, depending on the expansion forces of the stent. With regular expansion pressure the mucosa between the struts becomes oedematous. This causes mucosal protrusions between the metal filaments that may coalesce later.[75] The mucosa around the struts is damaged by the stent. In a reparative attempt, granulation tissue develops that may cover the whole stent in a matter of weeks.[76] With time, granulation tissue becomes less pronounced and squamous metaplastic epithelium develops, finally covering the stent. This epithelium has fewer cilia than normal respiratory epithelium. None the less, it may be capable of transporting mucus and secretions, enabling a mucosal clearance.[77]

When the compression forces exerted by the stent are excessive, they may cause ulceration and pressure necrosis involving deeper layers. These changes may even affect surrounding structures, for example the oesophagus or neighbouring vessels.[78,79]

Non-bacterial inflammatory changes may be observed in the respiratory epithelium and the submucosa. In the presence of microorganisms the events are modified. If a metal stent becomes colonized by bacteria, its incorporation in any form of tissue is precluded (e.g. in the tracheobronchial system, gastrointestinal system or urinary tract). Even though there may be apparent coverage of the stent surface, histology shows that there are still mucosal cells on the abluminal side of the stent.[52,80]

When placed in areas or wound surfaces damaged by prior manipulation, the stent will initially become covered by mucus, cell detritus and necrotic material. This may originate from the underlying disease or be the result of the manipulation. In tumorous areas, this cover may be all that is observed in the beginning. Later, tumour may grow through the interstices between the stent struts, leading to stent occlusion. However, occlusion is sometimes also caused by excessive granulation tissue.

Stents in the ureter and urethra

Ureter

When these stents are placed in the ureter, there are papillary mucosal proliferations between the struts; these can be seen endoscopically as papillary projections.[81] With excessive stent diameters, these proliferations have been reported to be more pronounced; this, however, is not universally accepted.[82,83]

With time, stents are lined (and frequently occluded) by a firmer and smoother layer of tissue.[81] When this is debrided mechanically, an underlying confluent flattened appearance becomes evident. The findings on histological examination in such cases are variable, depending, in part, on the underlying disease. Mixtures of hyperplastic urothelium and granulation tissue, or transitional cell carcinoma and granulation tissue, have been observed. Even after stent incorporation into the ureteric wall, the stimulus for the hyperplastic response is still active. In addition to reactive inflammation, fibrosis and tumour growth, the resulting mucosal hyperplasia is one of the factors responsible for the frequently observed rapid occlusion of metallic stents in the ureter.[81]

Urethra

When bare metal stents are placed in the urethra, the struts are at least partially covered by the longitudinal folds of mucosa.[84] The connective tissue core in some of the folds becomes oedematous. Numerous dilated capillaries and diffuse infiltration of lymphoid cells in these folds may be detected; sometimes, multifocal haemorrhage is observed. With stent diameters not exceeding 1.3 times the urethral dimensions, only a mild inflammatory infiltrate is seen. While there is no epithelial overgrowth of the stent wire if struts are thick – e.g. with

Gianturco stents (Cook Inc., Bloomington, IN, USA) – Wallstent endoprostheses in canine urethra are partially covered by epithelial overgrowth.[85]

References

1   Schultz JS, Lindenauer SM, Penner JA, Barenberg S. Determinants of thrombus formation on surfaces. *Trans Am Soc Artif Intern Organs* 1980; **26**: 279.

2   Wilentz IR, Sanborn TA, Haudenschild CC, Valeri CR, Ryan TJ, Faxon DP. Platelet accumulation in experimental angioplasty: time course and relation to vascular injury. *Circulation* 1987; **75**: 636–642.

3   Salam TA, Taylor B, Suggs WD, Hanson SR, Lumsden AB. Reaction to injury following balloon angioplasty and intravascular stent placement in the canine femoral artery. *Am Surg* 1994; **60**: 353–357.

4   Palmaz JC. Intravascular stents: Tissue–stent interactions and design considerations. *AJR* 1993; **160**: 613–618.

5   DePalma VA, Baier RE, Ford JW, Gott VL, Furuse A. Investigation of three surface properties of several metals and their relationship to blood compatibility. *J Biomed Mater Res* 1972; **3**: 37–75.

6   Sawyer PN, Page JW. Bio-electric phenomena as an etiologic factor in intravascular thrombosis. *Am J Physiol* 1953; **175**: 103.

7   Palmaz JC, Sibbitt RR, Reuter SR, Tio FO, Rice WJ. Expandable intraluminal graft: a preliminary study. *Radiology* 1985; **156**: 73–77.

8   Palmaz JC, Sprague EA. Basic interactions at the prosthetic blood interface. In: Liermann D, (ed.) *Stents – State of the art and future developments*. Morin Heights, Canada: Polyscience Publ. Inc., 1995.

9   Strecker EP, Liermann D, Barth KH *et al.* Expandable tubular stents for treatment of arterial occlusive disease: experimental and clinical results. *Radiology* 1990; **175**: 97–101.

10 Barth KH, Virmanni R, Strecker EP *et al.* Flexible tantalum stents implanted in aortas and iliac arteries: effects in normal canines. *Radiology* 1990; **175**: 91–96.

11 Nöldge G, Richter GM, Siegerstetter V, Garcia O, Palmaz JC. Tierexperimentelle Untersuchungen über den Einfluß der Flußrestriktion auf die Thrombogenität des Palmaz-Stentes mittels 111 Indium-markierter Thrombozyten. *Fortschr Röntgenstr* 1990; **152**: 264.

12 Bair RE, Dutton RC. Initial events in interaction of blood with foreign surface. *J Biomed Mater Res* 1969; **3**: 191–206.

13 Schatz RA, Palmaz JC, Tio FO, Garcia O, Reuter SR. Balloon-expandable intracoronary stent in the adult dog. *Circulation* 1987; **76**: 450–457.

14 Tominaga R, Emoto H, Kambic H, Harasaki H, Jikua T, Nose Y. Intravascular endoprostheses. Effect of surface geometry on restenosis and side branch patency. *Trans Am Soc Artif Intern Organs* 1989; **35**: 376–378.

15 Schatz RA, Palmaz JC, Tio F, Garcia O. Report of a new radiopaque balloon expandable stent (RBEIS) in canine coronary arteries. *Circulation* 1988; **78**(Suppl. II): II–448.

16 Palmaz JC, Kopp DT, Hayashi H *et al.* Normal and stenotic renal arteries: experimental balloon-expandable intraluminal stenting. *Radiology* 1987; **164**: 705–708.

17 Duprat G Jr, Wright KC, Charnsangavej C, Wallace S, Gianturco C. Self-expanding metallic stents for small vessels: an experimental evaluation. *Radiology* 1987; **162**: 469–472.

18 Schild H. Stent-Implantation-Grundlagen Pathophysiologie, Mechanik, medikamentöse Zusatztherapie. In: Friedmann G, Gross-Fengels W, Neufang K (eds) *Stent-Implantation und vaskuläre MR-Diagnostik*. Berlin: Springer-Verlag, 1991; 101–110.

19 Brown CH, Lemuth RF, Hellums JD, Leverett LB, Alfrey CP. Response of human platelets to shear stress *Trans Am Soc Artif Intern Organs* 1975; **21**: 35–39.

20 Stemerman MB, Spaet T, Pitlick F, Cintron J, Lejnicks I, Tiell ML. Intimal healing. *Am J Pathol* 1977; **87**: 125.

21 Birinyi LK, LoGerfo LW. Intimal hyperplasia: evolving concepts of pathophysiology and therapy. *Perspect Vasc Surg* 1989; **2**: 97–111.

22 Chesebro JH, Lam JYT, Badimon L, Fuster V. Restenosis after arterial angioplasty: a hemorrheologic response to injury. *Am J Cardiol* 1987; **60**: 10B–16B.

23 Rousseau H, Puel J, Joffre F *et al.* Self expanding endovascular prosthesis: an experimental study. *Radiology* 1987; **164**: 709–714.

24 Majesky MW, Reidy MA, Bowen-Pope DF *et al.* PDGF ligand and receptor gene expression during repair of arterial injury. *J Cell Biol* 1990; **111**: 2149–2158.

25 Sitaras NM, Sariban E, Pantazis P, Zetter B, Antoniades HN. Human iliac artery endothelial cells express both genes encoding the chains of platelet derived growth factor (PDGF) and synthesize PDGF-like mitogen. *J Cell Physiol* 1987; **132**: 376-380.

26 Ferns GA, Raines EW, Sprugel KH *et al.* Inhibition of neointimal smooth muscle accumulation after angioplasty by an antibody to PDGF. *Science* 1991; **253**: 1129–1132.

27 Karas SP, Gravanis MB, Santoian EC, Robinson KA, Anderberg KA, King SB III. Coronary intimal proliferation after balloon injury and stenting in swine: an animal model of restenosis. *J Am Coll Cardiol* 1992; **20**: 467–474.

28 Consigny PM, Tulenko TN, Nicosia RF. Immediate and long term effects of angioplasty on normal rabbit iliac artery. *Arteriosclerosis* 1986; **6**: 265–276.

29 Lindner V, Lappi Da Baird A, Majack RA, Reidy MA. Role of basic fibroblast growth factor in vascular lesion formation. *Circ Res* 1991; **68**: 106–113.

30 Robinson KA, Roubin G, King S, Siegel R, Rodgers G, Apkarian RP. Correlated microscopic observations of arterial responses to intravascular stenting. *Scan Microsc* 1989; **3**: 665–679.

31 Palmaz JC, Tio FO, Schatz RA, Alvarado R, Rees C, Garcia FS. Early endothelialization of balloon-expandable stents: experimental observations. *J Intervent Radiol* 1988; **3**: 119–124.

32 Palmaz JC, Windeler SA, Garcia F *et al.* Atherosclerotic rabbit aortas: expandable intraluminal grafting. *Radiology* 1986; **160**: 723–726.

33 Noishiki Y: Pattern of arrangement of smooth muscle cells in neointimae of synthetic vascula prostheses. *J Thorac Cardiovasc Surg* 1976; **75**: 894.

34 Roeren T. New therapeutic options for intimal hyperplasia. In: Liermann D (ed.) *Stents – state of the art and future developments*. Morin Heights, Canada: Polyscience Publ. Inc., 1995.

35 Ross R, Clomset JA, Kariya B, Harker LA. A platelet dependent factor that stimulates the proliferation of arterial smooth muscle cells in vitro. *Proc Natl Acad Sci USA* 1974; **71**: 1207.

36 Maass D, Demiere D, Deaton D, Largiader F. Transluminal implantation of self-adjusting expandable prosthesis: principles, techniques and results. *Prog Artif Organs* 1983; **2**: 979.

37 Wright KC, Wallace S, Charnsangavej C, Carrasco H, Gianturco C. Percutaneous intravascular stents: an experimental evaluation. *Radiology* 1985; **156**: 69.

38 Zollikofer CL, Largiader I, Bruhlmann WF *et al.* Endovascular stenting of veins and grafts: preliminary clinical experience. *Radiology* 1988; **167**: 707.

39 Zollikofer CL, Reha F, Bruhlmann W *et al.* Acute and long-term effects of massive balloon dilatation on the aortic wall and vasa vasorum. *Radiology* 1987; **164**: 145–149.

40 Beyar R, Shofti R, Grenedier E *et al.* Coronary arterial histological response to the self expandable nitinol stent. *J Am Coll Cardiol* 1993; **21**(2): 336 A.

41 Beyar R, Shofti R, Grenedier E, Henry M, Globerman O, Beyar M. Self-expandable nitinol stent for cardiovascular applications: canine and human experience. *Cathet Cardiovasc Diagn* 1994; **32**: 162–170.

42 Hehrlein C, Zimmermann M, Pill J, Metz J, Kübler W, von Hodenberg E. The role of elastic recoil after balloon angioplasty of rabbit arteries and its prevention by stent implantation. *Eur Heart J* 1994; **15**: 277–280.

43 Schwartz SM, Campbell GR, Campbell JH. Replication of smooth muscle cells in vascular disease. *Circ Res* 1986; **58**: 427.

44 Schatz RA. A view of vascular stents. *Circulation* 1989; **79**: 445–457.

45 Sigwart U, Puel J, Mirkovitch V, Joffre F, Kappenberger L. Intravascular stents to prevent occlusion and restenosis after transluminal angioplasty. *N Engl J Med* 1987; **316**: 701.

46 Fontaine AB, Spigos DG, Eaton G *et al.* Stent-induced intimal hyperplasia: are there fundamental differences between flexible and rigid stent designs? *J Vasc Intervent Radiol* 1994; **5**: 739–744.

47 Faxon DP, Sanborn TA, Haudenschild CC, Ryan TJ. Effect of antiplatelet therapy on restenosis after experimental angioplasy. *Am J Cardiol* 1984; **53**: 72c.

48 Rodgers GP, Minor ST, Robinson K *et al.* Adjuvant therapy for intracoronary stents. *Circulation* 1990; **82**: 560.

49 Fischell TA, Abbas MA, Kallmann RF. Low-dose radiation inhibits clonal proliferation of smooth muscle cells: a new approach to restenosis. *Arterioscler Thromb* 1991; **11**: 1435 A.

50 Fischell RE, Fischell DR, Fischell TA. The potential of a beta particle-emitting stent to inhibit restenosis following catheter based revascularization: work in progress. In: Liermann D (ed.) *Stents – State of the art and future developments*. Morin Heights, Canada: Polyscience Publ. Inc., 1995.

51 Liermann D, Bottcher HD, Kollath J *et al.* Prophylactic endovascular radiotherapy to prevent intimal hyperplasia after stent implantation in femoropopliteal arteries. *Cardiovasc Intervent Radiol* 1994; **17**: 12–16.

52 Gristina AG. Biomaterial centered infection: microbiological adhesion versus tissue integration. *Science* 1987; **237**: 1588–1595.

53 Garratt K, Holmes D, Schwartz R, Camrud A, Jorgenson M. Balloon dilatation of restenotic lesions within metallic coronary stents. Initial clinical and histopathologic observations. *J Am Coll Cardiol* 1992; **19**: 109 A.

54 Macander PJ, Roubin GS, Agrawal SK, Cannon AD, Dean LS, Baxley WA. Balloon angioplasty for treatment of in-stent restenosis: feasability, safety and efficacy. *Cathet Cardiovasc Diagn* 1994; **32**: 125–131.

55 King SB III. Vascular stents and atherosclerosis. *Circulation* 1989; **79**: 460–462.

56 Vorwerk D, Redha F, Neuerburg J, Clerc C, Günther RW. Neointima formation following arterial placement of self-expanding stents of different radial force: experimental results. *Cardiovasc Intervent Radiol* 1994; **17**: 27–32.

57 Zollikofer CL, Largiader I, Bruhlmann WF *et al.* Endovascular stenting of veins and grafts: preliminary clinical experience. *Radiology* 1988; **167**: 707.

58 Pisco JM, Correia M, Esperanca-Pina J, de Sousa LA. Microcirculatory changes following stenting. In: Liermann D (ed.) *Stents – State of the art and future developments.* Morin Heights, Canada: Polyscience Publ. Inc., 1995.

59 Pisco J, Correia M, Esperanca-Pina J, de Sousa LA. Vasa vasorum changes following stent placement in experimental arterial stensoses. *J Vasc Intervent Radiol* 1993; **4**: 269–273.

60 Back M, Kopschok G, Müller M, Cavaye D, Donayre C, White AR. Changes in arterial wall compliance after endovascular stenting. *J Vasc Surg* 1994; **19**: 905–911.

61 Leung DYM, Glagon S, Methews MD. Cyclic stretching stimulates synthesis of matrix components by arterial smooth muscle cells in vitro. *Science* 1976; **191**: 475–477.

62 Baird RN, Abbott WM. Pulsatile blood flow in arterial grafts. *Lancet* 1976; **2**: 948–949.

63 Abbott WM, Megerman J, Hasson JE, L Tralien G, Warnock DF. Effect of compliance mismatch on vascular graft patency. *J Vasc Surg* 1987: **5**: 376–382.

64 Okuhn SP, Conelly DP, Calakos C, Ferell L, Man Xiang P, Goldstone J. Does compliance mismatch alone cause neointimal hyperplasia? *J Vasc Surg* 1989; **9**: 35.

65 Palmaz JC, Sibbitt RR, Reuter STR, Garcia F, Tio FO. Expandable intrahepatic portocaval shunt stents: early experience in the dog. *AJR* 1985; **145**: 821–825.

66 Kerlan RK, LaBerge JM, Gordon RL, Ring EJ. Transjugular intrahepatic portosystemic shunts: current status. *AJR* 1995; **164**: 1059–1066.

67 LaBerge JM, Ferrel LB, Ring EJ. Histopathologic study of transjugular intrahepatic portosystemic shunts. *J Vasc Intervent Radiol* 1991; **2**: 549–556.

68 LaBerge JM, Ferell LD, Ring EJ, Gordon RL. Histopathology of TIPS stenosis and occlusions. *J Vasc Intervent Radiol* 1993; **4**: 779–786.

69 Kichikawa K, Nishida N, Uchida BT, Timmermans HA, Keller FS, Rösch J. Animal model for pseudointimal hyperplasia in TIPS. In: SCVIR 18th annual scientific meeting programme. Fairfax, USA: *Soc Cardiovasc Intervent Radiol* 1993: 96.

70 Zemel G, Katzen BT, Becker GJ, Benenati JF, Sallee D. Percutaneous transjugular portosystemic shunt. *JAMA* 1991; **17**: 390–393.

71 Murphy KD, Encarnacion CE, Le VA, Palmaz JC. Iliac artery stent placement with the Palmaz stent: follow up study. *J Vasc Intervent Radiol* 1995; **65**: 321–329.

72 Redha F, Zollikofer CL, Uhlschmid GK *et al.* Combination of angioplasty and intraarterial stent: an experimental study. *Radiology* 1987; **165**: 309.

73 Vorwerk D, Kissinger G, Handt S, Günther RW. Long term patency of Wallstent endoprostheses in benign biliary obstructions: experimental results. *J Vasc Intervent Radiol* 1993; **4**: 625–634.

74 Carrasco H, Wallace S, Charnsangavej C *et al.* Expandable biliary endoprosthesis: an experimental study. *AJR* 1985; **145**: 1279–1281.

75 Rauber K, Franke C, Seyd Ali S, Bensmann G. Experimentelle Erfahrungen mit Nitinol Prothesen. In : Kollath J, Liermann D (eds) *Stents*. Konstanz: Schnetzor Verlag, 1990: 65–70.

76 Wallace S, Charnsangavej C, Ogawa K *et al.* Tracheobronchial tree: expandable metallic stents used in experimental and clinical applications. *Radiology* 1986; **158**: 309–312.

77 Grewe P, Krampe K, Müller K-M., Becker H-D. Makroskopische und histomorphologische Veränderungen der Bronchialwand nach der Implantation von Nitinol-Stents. In: Kollath J, Liermann D (eds) *Stents III*. Konstanz: Schnetzor Verlag, 1995: 245–249.

78 Vinograd I, Klin B, Brosh T, Weinberg M, Flomenblit Y, Nevo Z. A new intratracheal stent made from nitinol, an alloy with 'shape memory effect'. *J Thorac Cardiovasc Surg* 1994; **107**: 1255–1261.

79 Loeff DS, Filler RM, Gorenstein A *et al.* A new tracheobronchial reconstruction: experimental and clinical studies. *J Pediatr Surg* 1988; **23**: 1113–1117.

80 Alvarado R, Palmaz JC, Garcia Oj, Tio FO, Rees CR. Evaluation of polymer-coated balloon expandable stents in bile ducts. *Radiology* 1989; **170**: 975–978.

81 Pollak JS, Rosenblatt MM, Egglin TK, Dickey KW, Glickman M. Treatment of ureteral obstructions with the Wallstent endoprosthesis: preliminary results. *J Vasc Intervent Radiol* 1995; **6**: 417–425.

82 Millward SF, Thijssen Am, Mariner JR, Moors DE, Mai KT. Effect of a metallic balloon expanded stent on normal rabbit ureter. *J Vasc Intervent Radiol* 1991; **2**: 557–650.

83 Wright KC, Dobben RL, Magal C, Ogawa K, Wallace S, Gianturco C. Occlusive effect of metallic stents on canine ureters. *Cardiovasc Intervent Radiol* 1983; **16**: 230–240.

84 Dobben RL, Wright KC, Dolenz K, Wallace S, Gianturco C. Prostatic urethra dilatation with the Gianturco self expanding metallic stent: a feasibility study in cadaver specimens and dogs. *AJR* 1991; **156**: 757–761.

85 Milroy EJG, Cooper JE, Wallsten H *et al.* A new treatment for urethral strictures. *Lancet* 1988; **1**: 1424–1427.

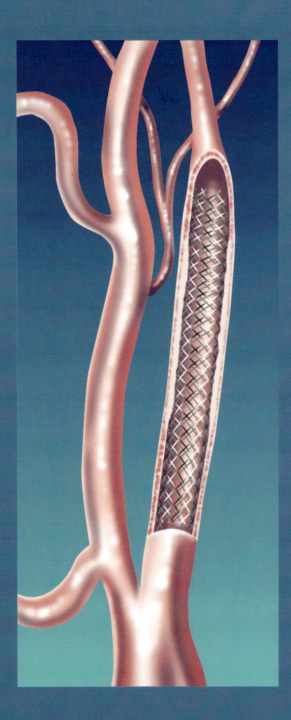

Chapter 10

Stent placement in arteriosclerotic disease of the internal carotid artery

K. Mathias

Introduction

Percutaneous transluminal angioplasty (PTA) of the carotid artery began in 1977 with animal experiments and in 1979 when a 32-year-old female patient with fibromuscular dysplasia causing symptomatic carotid stenosis was treated for the first time by balloon angioplasty.[1–3] Shortly afterwards, other types of non-atherosclerotic stenoses of the carotid artery were successfully handled by PTA.[4–11]

Clinical symptoms in atherosclerotic carotid stenosis are caused by embolic disease in more than 80% of patients and in less than 20% by haemodynamic impairment of cerebral circulation. Therefore, the main aim of invasive treatment is the removal of plaque material, to prevent a further and ultimately damaging embolism. PTA of atherosclerotic carotid stenosis was considered unsuitable for a cure of the disease because the atherosclerotic deposits are not removed by this method. Moreover, the risks of cerebral artery embolism and thrombosis were considered unacceptable by many. Therefore, techniques of protecting the carotid artery with balloons and washout to prevent embolism were discussed.[17]

The first patients with atherosclerotic disease were successfully treated by PTA from 1980 onwards.[5,11–14] Only patients with smoothly delineated sandglass-like carotid stenosis in multiple vessels, who were poor candidates for surgery and suffered from haemodynamic impairment of the cerebral circulation, were selected. However, certain disadvantages of simple balloon angioplasty turned out to be a severe obstacle to general acceptance of the method; these included:

- heterogenous material at the carotid bifurcation[15] (atherosclerotic debris, subintimal haematoma, thrombus, calcification)
- residual stenosis after PTA[16]
- intimal cracking, flap formation and dissection[17]
- risk of embolism[18]
- unknown early and late outcome
- the simplicity of carotid surgery
- the decreasing complication rate of carotid surgery.

The unwillingness of vascular surgeons and neurologists in many centres to refer patients for PTA, and the lack of quantitative data on complications and results of carotid PTA, slowed down the development of the method. It was not possible to collect data from several centres and to establish knowledge of internal carotid artery PTA in order to determine the feasibility, indications and efficacy of this intervention.

In 1989, a stent was placed for the first time in the internal carotid artery when the control angiogram revealed an intimal flap after PTA and an improvement of the PTA result became necessary.[16,17] The procedure was well tolerated and the patient continues to have a good long-term result, with a patent artery and no recurrent stenosis after 7 years.

Choice of stent

Several types of stent are currently available but some are more appropriate than others for use in the carotid arteries. The required characteristics are defined by the exposed position of the carotid artery, and the bending of the vessel with each movement of the head. The fact that the pathological process is most commonly located at the carotid bifurcation also must be considered as this requires stent placement in vessels with different diameters (Table 10.1).

The internal diameter of the internal carotid artery varies from 5 to 7 mm and the mean diameter is 5.7 mm. The common carotid artery measures 7–10 mm. When the stent is placed across the bifurcation, it has to adapt itself to arteries of different diameters. The stent should be in contact with the vessel wall in order for it to be covered by a neointima. All these requirements are best met by the Wallstent™ (Schneider, Minneapolis, MN, USA). Its narrow meshwork is useful in preventing embolism during balloon dilatation. Balloon-expandable stents should not be used in the carotid artery because they all tend to collapse. This phenomenon has been observed even with the fairly stiff Palmaz™ stent (Johnson & Johnson Interventional Systems, Warren, NJ, USA).

The appropriate diameter and length of the stent depend on the dimensions of the common carotid artery and the extent of the stenosis. The stent should fit the common carotid artery closely to achieve good healing and formation of a flat neointima that will prevent thrombus deposition at that site (Fig. 10.1). The most commonly used stent diameter is 8 mm. A stent length from 20 to 32 mm is sufficient in most patients. In dilated common carotid arteries 10 mm stents often need to be used; 45 mm long stents may be necessary in extended disease involving the proximal common or the distal internal carotid artery. When the stenosis is restricted to the internal carotid artery and more than 5 mm away from the bifurcation, a stent with a diameter of 6 mm can be applied, thus obviating the need to cross the orifice of the external carotid artery.

- self-expandable
- flexible
- non-collapsing
- no interruption of blood flow during placement
- low thrombogenicity
- narrow meshwork
- tapering
- sonographically transparent

Table 10.1

Properties of stents for carotid placement

Figure 10.1 (a)
A 64-year-old man with TIAs: (a) >90% stenosis of the left internal carotid artery (ICA) with poor opacification of the distal ICA. (b) After stent PTA normal diameter of the ICA; slight spastic reaction distal to the site of the stent.

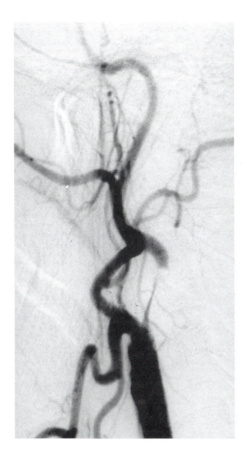

(b)

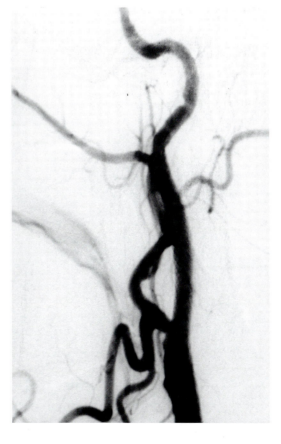

Technique of stent placement

Stents can be placed in the internal carotid artery before or after balloon dilatation. Initially, secondary stent placement was used to improve the dilatation result when the control angiogram revealed residual stenosis of more than 50%, intimal flap or dissection. There was a 20% rate of residual stenosis after PTA in 241 cases: in 52% this was related to underdilatation, with small balloons, in an effort to minimize the incidence of major plaque rupture and embolization. Later on, primary stent placement was preferred in order to reduce the rate of embolization during dilatation. In tight rigid stenoses predilatation with a 3–4 mm balloon may become necessary to pass the narrowed artery segment with the stent catheter.

After angiographic documentation, the stenosis is probed with a steerable guidewire with a floppy tip (0.021 in), and a diagnostic catheter with a sidewinder or vertebral curve configuration. In irregular ulcerated stenoses sometimes a J-curved Terumo® guidewire (0.035 in) is helpful. The guidewire should be long enough for catheter exchange. The stent catheter is introduced and advanced to the stenosis via a 7 Fr sheath at the groin. In elongated iliac arteries a long sheath is used, with the tip in the abdominal aorta, or a guiding catheter in the common carotid artery.

The road map technique is helpful in exact positioning of the stent, which otherwise might be difficult because of the considerable shortening of the Wallstent after deployment and dilatation within the stent. The stent is released only partially and its position is checked using a single exposure. It can be pulled back should it be advanced too far, but it cannot be pushed forward when the lesion is not covered completely. Therefore, it is better to place the stent delivery catheter far enough distally when the ideal position is not certain because correction of the stent position is then still possible with a partially deployed stent. When the stent is completely released, its radial force reduces the degree of stenosis. The stent delivery catheter is now exchanged for a dilatation catheter and the stenosis is dilated with the balloon (Fig. 10.2) During all these manoeuvres the guidewire is kept in place to allow easy access to the stenosis. The guidewire should not be moved too much after crossing the stenosis, to avoid a sawing effect on the plaque. When a guiding catheter is used and is advanced to the common carotid artery, it is safer to direct the guidewire into the external carotid artery before the catheter is pushed into the common carotid artery.

Monitoring

Continuous pressure monitoring is useful and facilitates registration of the pressure gradient before and after dilatation. When the poststenotic pressure (back pressure) is reduced to less than 60 mmHg, the risk of a possible ischaemic event is increased and special care is necessary. During stent PTA, electrocardiography should be used to observe changes of heart rate. Severe bradycardia may occur and may be accompanied by a decrease in blood pressure. Equipment for pacing and defibrillation should be readily available. Additional monitoring techniques are transcranial Doppler ultrasound, conventional and on-line Fourier transformed electroencephalography and brainstem auditory-evoked potentials. In stent PTA of carotid arteries these methods are particularly useful

Figure 10.2
Stent PTA with primary stenting. (a) Guidewire in the ICA; the stent has just been deployed and shows a typical constriction at the site of the stenosis. (b) 6 mm balloon is inflated; (c) stent has opened completely.

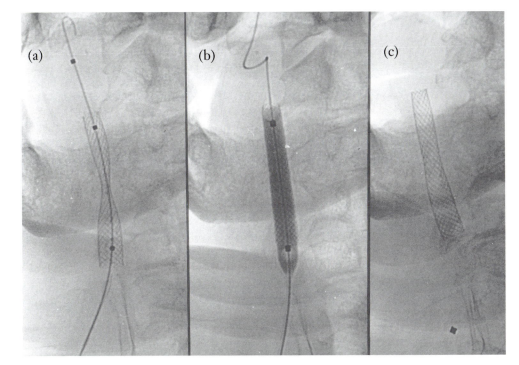

in answering scientific questions, e.g. rate of microembolism, but are not mandatory, and prolong the treatment time. However, such neuromonitoring is valuable in local fibrinolysis of thrombotic cerebral artery disease requiring an infusion time of several hours.

Medication

Before stent placement and dilatation the patient receives a premedication with 0.5–1.0 mg atropine according to his or her heart rate. If the carotid body is stimulated by the stent or balloon during balloon dilatation, atropine helps to prevent severe bradycardia. In addition, the patient is given 10,000 U heparin and 5 mg nifedipine. For 2 days after the intervention 25,000 U heparin and 300 mg aspirin are given. In cases of sensitivity to aspirin, 250 mg tyclipidine are given twice daily.

Indications (Table 10.2)

The main indication for stent PTA is carotid stenosis exceeding 70% (Fig. 10.3).[18,19] This is supported by the results of surgical studies, especially the North American Study of Carotid Endarterectomy (NASCET), the European Carotid Surgery Trial (ECST) and the Asymptomatic Carotid Surgery Trial (ACST).[20-2] The clinical stage of the patients is not so important because patients with severe stenosis have nearly the same annual stroke incidences of 5–7% in stages I and II.[23] Nearly 80% of the author's patients were in stage II (Fig. 10.4). In stage IV he recommends stent PTA when a high-degree stenosis is responsible for recurring transient ischaemic attacks (TIAs) and when the infarcted area is small.

Stage I	Atherosclerotic stenosis > 70%
Stage II	Atherosclerotic stenosis > 70%
Stage II (imminent stroke)	Atherosclerotic stenosis > 70%
Stage IV	Atherosclerotic stenosis > 70%; small infarcted area
Postoperative recurrence	Stenosis > 70%
Spontaneous dissection	Internal carotid artery not occluded
After PTA	Dissection after PTA of fibromuscular dysplasia

Table 10.2
Indications for stent PTA

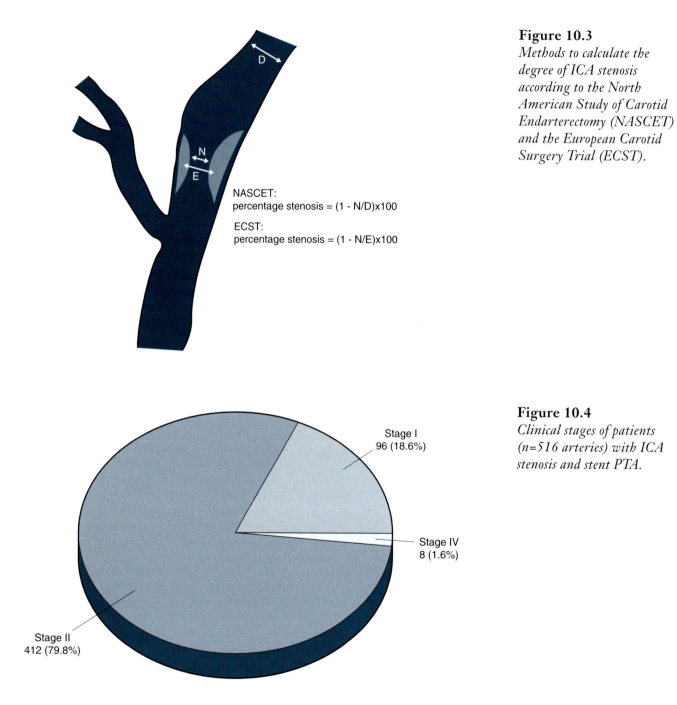

NASCET:
percentage stenosis = (1 - N/D)x100

ECST:
percentage stenosis = (1 - N/E)x100

Figure 10.3
Methods to calculate the degree of ICA stenosis according to the North American Study of Carotid Endarterectomy (NASCET) and the European Carotid Surgery Trial (ECST).

Stage I
96 (18.6%)

Stage IV
8 (1.6%)

Stage II
412 (79.8%)

Figure 10.4
Clinical stages of patients (n=516 arteries) with ICA stenosis and stent PTA.

These patients are at risk of developing a new stroke, which might disable them more severely or might even lead to death. Acute crescendo ischaemia stroke may be prevented by stent PTA.[24] Recurrent stenosis of the carotid artery after surgical treatment is an appropriate indication for stent PTA.

The indications for stent PTA are almost independent of the morphology of the stenosis. Irregular surface, thrombus or ulcerations are no reasons to refrain from the intervention. However, thick circular or horseshoe-like calcifications are relative contraindications for stent PTA because overdistention of the non-calcified segment of the arterial circumference may cause a false aneurysm or even rupture of the vessel. In such cases the degree and location of calcifications should be examined by spiral CT before stent PTA is attempted.[25]

Experience and results

In a series of 516 atherosclerotic stenoses of the internal carotid artery in 480 patients, stent PTA has been performed in 275 and simple balloon angioplasty in 241 with a success rate of 99% (Fig. 10.5). The mean age was 61 years with a range of 49–88 years. Patients with bilateral disease, (n = 36) were treated on both sides in one or two sessions. In 27 arteries, stents were used in an effort to improve the result of balloon dilatation (secondary stenting). A total of 248 carotid arteries were treated by primary stenting with subsequent PTA within the stent (Fig. 10.6 and Fig. 10.7). In a very small number of cases, predilatation of the stenosis with an undersized balloon was necessary to pass a tight stenosis with the catheter.

In patients with occluded iliac arteries or elongated supra-aortic vessels, stents could be placed using an axillary approach. In most of the patients in the stent group, primary stenting (248/275) was carried out. In nearly all patients, predilatation of the stenosis before stent placement proved unnecessary. Only in

Figure 10.5
Distribution of interventions between ICA PTA and stent PTA (n=516 arteries).

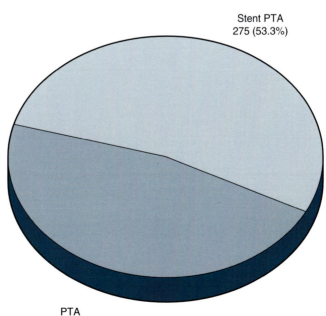

Stent PTA
275 (53.3%)

PTA
241 (46.7%)

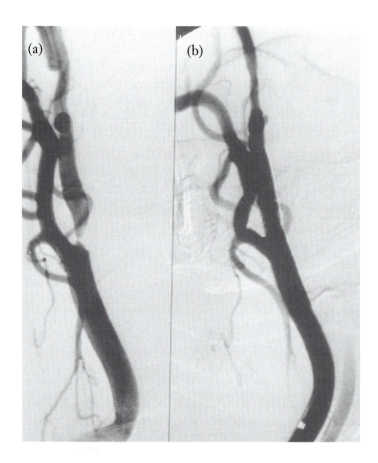

Figure 10.6
68-year-old man with TIAs and a small infarction in the middle cerebral artery territory. (a) Short stenosis of the left ICA >90%. (b) Stenosis completely removed after stent PTA.

Figure 10.7
72-year-old woman with TIAs. (a) Atherosclerosis of the carotid bifurcation with ulceration of the CCA, 75% stenosis of the ICA and 60% stenosis of the ECA. (b) After stent PTA, normal width of the ICA. (c) Control angiogram after 6 months: unchanged appearance, with a thin layer of neointima.

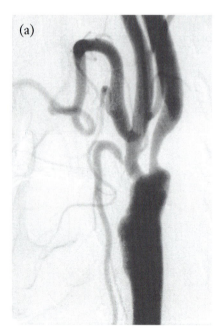
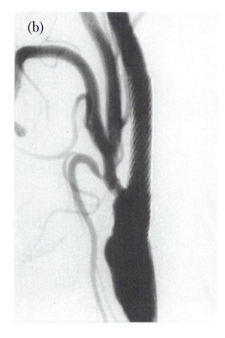
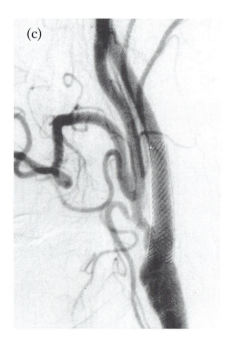

patients in whom the stenosis could not be crossed easily was pre-dilatation with an undersized balloon (diameter 4 mm) performed. This was done in order to prevent a situation where the stent catheter cannot be extracted after deployment of the stent without pulling the stent back into the common carotid artery. When the hoop strength of the stent is not sufficient to widen the vessel and let the olive at the tip of the catheter pass through the stenosis, the problem described above many arise; this happened in only 6 of 275 patients (2.2%). In these cases it was necessary to fix the stent with aid of a second catheter introduced into the common carotid artery to enable the stent delivery catheter to be withdrawn without the stent.

The data of 247 of the 275 patients who were treated from July 1989 to August 1995 were evaluated with regard to early results, complications, degree of intimal proliferation, and long-term patency (Fig. 10.8). The follow-up information is summarized in Table 10.3.

Stent PTA was carried out successfully in 273 of 275 arteries (99.3%). In one patient with a dilated aortic arch and elongated internal carotid artery it was not possible to advance the stent catheter in the stenosis. After stent placement and PTA, a residual stenosis exceeding 20% was seen on angiography in only 6

Figure 10.8

Cumulative 3-year patency of the ICA after stent PTA (n=247 ICAs).

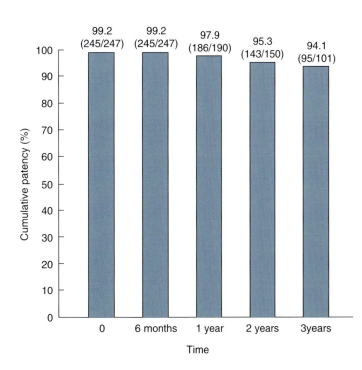

Table 10.3

Examinations before and after stent PTA of the internal carotid artery

Before stent PTA	Neurological examination
	Doppler ultrasound
	Magnetic resonance imaging (MRI) of the head
	Aortic arch and selective angiography
After stent PTA	Neurological examination
	Doppler ultrasound, repeated every 3 months
	MRI head within 48 hours after the intervention
	Selective angiography after 6 months

patients (6 of 273; 2.2%). In 267 patients the angiogram revealed an internal carotid artery of normal diameter and smooth contours. On cerebral angiography there was improved cerebral arterial flow in all patients. The cross-flow from the contralateral side via the anterior communicating artery disappeared in all cases.

In 7 patients deep ulcerations or false aneurysms were treated by placement of an uncovered stent (Fig. 10.9 and Fig. 10.10). Within 6 months, 6 of the 7 aneurysms had disappeared. In 1 patient the size of the aneurysm had diminished, but it was still visible. Haemodynamic repair – that is to say, reduction of lateral pressure and increased shear forces on the aneurysm by stent-related longitudinal direction of the bloodstream – seems to be sufficient in most patients with aneurysm formation. Treatment with covered stents is probably indicated only in exceptionally large aneurysms.

During the follow-up period 4 carotid arteries became occluded; 2 of the 4 patients suffered a stroke. Occlusion occurred 4 days, and 9, 10, and 32 months after the procedure. Recurrent stenoses of varying degree were observed (Table 10.4), requiring redilatation in one case. In all the other patients, only insignificant lumen reduction without haemodynamic effects was seen (Fig. 10.11).

Complications

Two types of complications occurred. An 84-year-old female patient developed signs of impaired fine motor control of a hand at the end of the intervention. Angiography showed some flow reduction in angular artery branches, but no embolic vessel occlusion could be detected. Regional fibrinolysis with 50 mg rt-PA was started immediately and followed by anticoagulation with 30,000 U heparin for 24 hours. Nevertheless, MRI revealed a small middle cerebral artery infarction. Four patients had a transient ischaemic attack within the first 4 hours

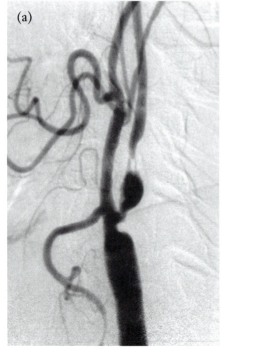

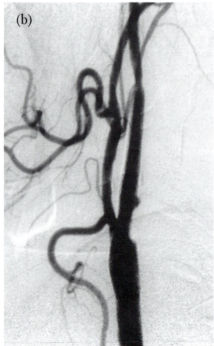

Figure 10.9
74-year-old man with TIAs of the left hemisphere.
(a) Complex stenosis: plaque of the CCA at the bifurcation, short 70% ICA stenosis, deep ulceration followed by a double-lumen >90% ICA stenosis. (b) After stent PTA slight residual stenosis of the CCA; poor opacification of the ICA ulcer which will completely disappear in a short time.

Figure 10.10
59-year-old man with TIAs of the right hemisphere. (a) ICA stenosis and two deep ulcerations (false aneurysm). (b) After stent PTA no opacification of the CCA ulcer and diminished filling of the larger distal aneurysm

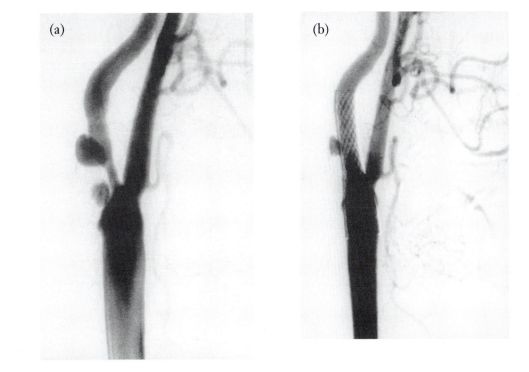

Table 10.4
Complications of stent PTA

Type	Number	Percentage
Stroke	1	0.36
Immediate TIA	4	1.45
Late TIA (<3 months)	1	0.36
Death	1	0.36
Total	7	2.54

Figure 10.11
68-year-old man with stent PTA 1 year previously. (a) Doppler sonography demonstrates a nearly normal flow pattern measured in the stented ICA segment. (b) The stent is well delineated in the CCA and ICA with a minimal waist at the ICA orifice; no significant myointimal hyperplasia.

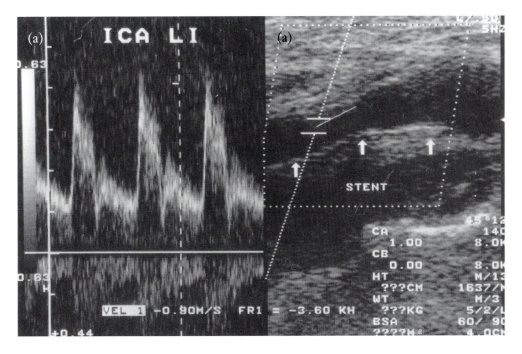

after the intervention. It is well known that, during carotid surgery and PTA, embolic signals can be detected by transcranial Doppler sonography during and after the procedure, but this phenomenon is clinically silent in most cases.[26] None of the author's patients required vascular surgery. One patient reported three recurrent TIAs within the first 3 months after stent PTA. After that period no further events occurred. At control angiography a smoothly delineated internal carotid artery of normal diameter was shown. Hospital mortality was low, with only one 82-year-old patient dying of myocardial infarction 5 days after stent PTA. During the follow-up period of up to 6 years, 2 strokes were recorded.

Myointimal hyperplasia

Growth of myointimal cells – so-called metabolically modified smooth muscle cells – is seen after vascular surgery, PTA and stent PTA, and presents a uniform reaction of an atherosclerotic arterial wall to the inflicted injury. Deposition of platelets and of neutrophils, as well as myointimal tissue growth, after stent placement is of special interest in coronary and peripheral arteries because a higher rate of recurrent stenosis may be expected in these vessels; by inference, the same applies to the internal carotid artery.[27] However, this assumption is unproven in the case of the internal carotid artery and the reaction of this artery to stent placement may differ from that of other arteries. The flow pattern of the internal carotid artery differs from that in other vessels with antegrade flow in systole as well as diastole. Cerebral perfusion and flow in the carotid artery are nearly constant throughout a wide range of blood pressures owing to the capacity for autoregulation of the cerebral circulation. Because of this constant blood flow the shear force applied to the vessel wall is weaker and less variable, and is probably accompanied by a less pronounced myointimal reaction. However, a foreign body in a pulsating artery that is bent with each movement of the head may favour the development of myointimal proliferation.

In order to obtain more information on the behaviour of the vessel wall after stent placement, Doppler ultrasound monitoring every 3 months and selective control angiography after 6 months were included in the follow-up protocol for all patients. Doppler ultrasound facilitated evaluation of the arterial lumen and the anterior wall of the stented common and internal carotid artery (Fig. 10.11); the posterior wall was not always seen clearly. The results of the control angiogram were relied on for the detection and quantification of myointimal hyperplasia. The data of 88 control angiograms are available for evaluation. The findings in three distinct groups are outlined in Table 10.5. Concentric or an eccentric narrowing of the arterial lumen was attributed to myointimal proliferation. When

Classification	Wall thickening (mm)	Arteries [n(%)]
No MIP	< 1	39 (44)*
Minor MIP	1–2	42 (48)
Major MIP	> 2	7 (8)

*This group of patients includes those with slight widening of the internal carotid artery.

Table 10.5
Classification and quantitative distribution of myointimal proliferation (MIP) in n = 88 arteries

the diameter of the internal carotid was normal (or even increased), but the stent was separated from the arterial lumen by 1–2 mm, this phenomenon was defined as stent ingrowth (Fig. 10.12 and Fig. 10.13). However, confirmation of this interpretation is not available.

Figure 10.12
Control angiogram 6 months after stent PTA of the ICA: no myointimal proliferation; only a thin neointima is seen.

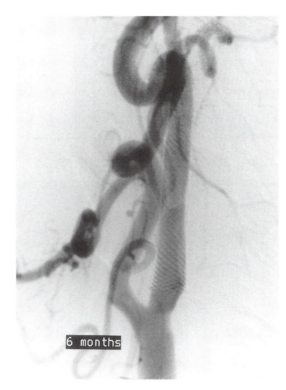

Figure 10.13
Control angiogram at 6 months: major myointimal proliferation (larger arrows); patent ECA.

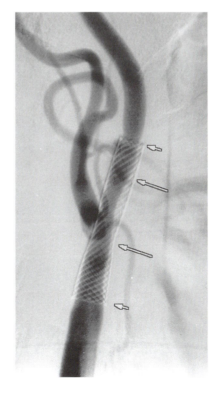

Stent ingrowth

In 28 patients the lumen of the internal carotid artery increased during the observation period. Moreover, the Wallstent was separated from the opacified inner surface of the arterial wall by 1–2 mm. Presumably, the constant hoop force of the Wallstent and the selection of a stent slightly wider than the arterial lumen are responsible for the widening of the arterial diameter as well as for the embedding of the stent in deeper layers of the vessel wall (Fig. 10.14). Atrophy of the media is observed especially where the struts of the stent cross over each other.[28] This pressure atrophy of the media may facilitate stent ingrowth, which is comparable to the ingrowth observed in other devices that apply a constant pressure to the vessel wall, such as caval filters, where the struts of the filter are deeply embedded in the venous wall.

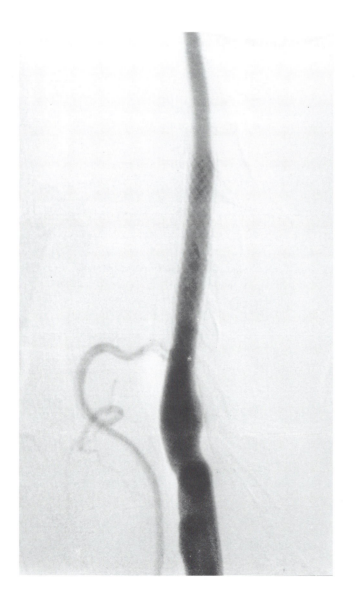

Figure 10.14
Control angiogram 6 months after stent PTA of the ICA: slight widening of the ICA lumen and stent ingrowth; the ECA was already occluded at the time of treatment.

Conclusions and outlook

Stent PTA has proved efficacious in the treatment of patients suffering from atherosclerotic stenosis of the internal carotid artery. It achieves better results than balloon angioplasty with regard to restoration of the arterial lumen and the smoothness of the vessel wall. The stent presumably influences the flow pattern at the bifurcation because the angle between the common carotid artery and the internal carotid artery is abolished, the axis of the vessel is straightened, and the bloodstream goes directly from the common carotid artery into the internal carotid artery. The importance of the changed haemodynamics is unknown, but may not be negligible. Without the usual shear forces at the bifurcation, the progress of the atherosclerotic process may differ from that with the normal anatomical arrangement or the situation after carotid surgery.[29]

The complication rate of carotid PTA is reduced further by stenting, placing this procedure in a competitive position with regard to vascular surgery. The European trial comparing thrombendarterectomy and PTA of the internal carotid artery in a prospectively randomized manner has shown no essential differences between the two methods during a period of more than 2 years. Considering the fact that the participating groups performing PTA are using an evolving technique, whereas vascular surgery has been established for 3 decades, these preliminary results are promising.[17,30] Stent PTA is now included in this trial and will probably lead to even better results. Nevertheless, it should be noted that stent PTA is not a generally applicable method of treatment, and should be performed only under trial conditions until further data regarding early and late outcome have become available.

Further development of stents will probably influence the technique during the next few years. The Wallstent is now improved and is more easily visible; this facilitates exact placement. Perhaps a stent with thinner struts and a narrower meshwork would be safer, because protrusion of atherosclerotic debris through the stent during PTA might be better prevented and the rate of embolism reduced. Many groups are working on coated stents, which should inhibit thrombus formation and myointimal proliferation. Covered stents are available, but must be improved. Perhaps covered stents will decrease the risk of embolization even more. However, before such stents are widely used it should be established whether occlusion of the external carotid artery – which is patent in most of the patients treated with a Wallstent – is well tolerated clinically. A great deal of scientific work in this field remains to be done.

References

1   Mathias K. Ein neuartiges Katheter-System zur perkutanen transluminalen Angioplastie von Karotisstenosen. *Fortschr Med* 1977; **95**: 1007–1011.

2   Mathias K, Mittermayer CH, Ensinger H, Neff W. Perkutane Katheterdilatation von Karotisstenosen. *ROFO* 1980; **133**: 258–261.

3   Mathias K. Perkutane transluminale Katheterbehandlung supraaortaler Arterienobstruktionen. *Angio* 1981; **3**: 47–50.

4   Hasso AN, Bird CR, Zinke DE, Thompson JR. Fibromuscular dysplasia of the internal carotid artery: percutaneous transluminal angioplasty. *AJR* 1981; **136**: 955–960.

5   Bockenheimer SA, Mathias K. Percutaneous transluminal angioplasty in arteriosclerotic internal carotid artery stenosis. *AJNR* 1983; **4**: 791–792.

6   Tievsky AL, Druy EM, Mardiat JG. Transluminal angioplasty in postsurgical stenosis of the extracranial carotid artery. *AJNR* 1983; **4**: 800–802.

7 Tisnado J, Vines FS, Barnes RW, Beachley MC, Cho SR. Percutaneous transluminal angioplasty following endarterectomy. *Radiology* 1984; **152**: 361–364.

8 Numaguchi Y, Puyau FA, Provenza LJ, Richardson DE. Percutaneous transluminal angioplasty of the carotid artery. Its application in post surgical stenosis. *Neuroradiology* 1984; **26**: 527–530.

9 Hodgins GW, Dutton JW. Transluminal dilatation for Takayasu's Arteritis. *Can J Surg* 1984; **27**: 355–357.

10 Courtheoux P, Theron J, Tournade A, Maiza D, Henriet JP, Braun JP. Percutaneous endoluminal angioplasty of post-endarterectomy carotid stenoses. *Neuroradiology* 1987; **29**: 186–189.

11 Theron J, Raymond J, Casasco A, Courtheoux P. Percutaneous angioplasty of atherosclerotic and postsurgical stenosis of carotid arteries. *AJNR* 1987; **8**: 495–500.

12 Mathias K, Bockenheimer S, von Reutern G, Heiss HW, Ostheim-Dzerowycz W. Katheterdilatation hirnversorgender Arterien. *Radiologe* 1983; **23**: 208–214.

13 Kachel R, Endert G, Basche S, Grossmann K, Glaser FH. Percutaneous transluminal angioplasty (dilatation) of carotid, vertebral, and innominate artery stenoses. *Cardiovasc Intervent Radiol* 1987; **10**: 142–146.

14 Kachel R. Percutaneous tranluminal angioplasty (PTA) of supra-aortic arteries especially of the carotid and vertebral artery. An alternative to vascular surgery? *J Mal Vasc* 1993; **18**: 254–257.

15 Hayward JK, Davies AH, Lamont PM. Carotid plaque morphology: a review. *Eur J Vasc Endovasc Surg* 1995; **9**: 368–374.

16 Mathias K. Percutaneous transluminal angioplasty in surpra-aortic artery disease. In: Roubin GS, Califf RM, O'Neill WW, Philips HR, Stack RS (eds). *Interventional Cardiovascular Medicine*. New York: Churchill Livingstone, 1994: 745–775.

17 Mathias K. Perkutane Rekanalisation der supreaaortalen und zerebralen Arterien. In: Günther RW, Thelen M (eds). *Interventionelle Radiologie*. Stuttgart: Thieme, 1996: 112–123.

18 Derauf BJ, Erickson DL, Castaneda-Zuniga WR, Cardella JF, Amplatz K. 'Washout' technique for brachiocephalic angioplasty. *AJR* 1986; **146**: 849–851.

19 Fox AJ. How to measure carotid stenosis. *Radiology* 1993; **186**: 316–318.

20 North American Symptomatic Carotid Endarterectomy Trial Collaborators. Beneficial effect of carotid endarterectomy in symptomatic patients with high-grade stenosis. *New Engl J Med* 1991; **325**: 445–453.

21 European Carotid Surgery Trialists' Collaborative Group. MRC European Carotid Surgery Trial: interim results for symptomatic patients with severe (70–99%) or with mild (0–29%) carotid stenosis. *Lancet* 1991; **337**(8752): 1235–1243.

22 Halliday AW, Thomas DJ, Mansfield AO. The asymptomatic carotid surgery trial (ACST). *Int Angiol* 1995; **14**: 18–20.

23 Executive Committee for the Asymptomatic Carotid Atherosclerosis Study. Endarterectomy for asymptomatic carotid artery stenosis. *JAMA* 1995; **273**: 1421–1428.

24 Shawl FA. Emergency percutaneous carotid stenting during stroke [letter]. *Lancet* 1995; **346**(8984): 1223.

25 Jaeger HJ, Goetz F, Kubasch M, Mathias K. Evaluation of atherosclerotic disease of the carotid bifurcation with spiral CT angiography. *Radiology* 1995; **197**(P): 144.

26 Markus HS, Clifton A, Buckenham T, Brown MM. Carotid angioplasty. Detection of embolic signals during and after the procedure. *Stroke* 1994; **25**: 2403–2406.

27 Parsson H, Cwikiel W, Johansson K, Swartbol P, Norgren L. Deposition of platelets and neutrophils in porcine iliac arteries after angioplasty and Wallstent placement compared with angioplasty alone. *Cardiovasc Intervent Radiol* 1994; **17**: 190–196.

28 Wakhloo AK, Tio FO, Lieber BB, Schellhammer F, Graf M, Hopkins LN. Self-expanding nitinol stents in canine vertebral arteries: hemodynamics and tissue response. *AJNR* 1995; **16**: 1043–1051.

29 Harrison MJG, Marshall J. Does the geometry of the carotid bifurcation affect its predisposition to atheroma? *Stroke* 1983; **14**: 117–123.

30 Marks MP, Dake MD, Steinberg GK, Norgash AM, Lane B. Stent placement for arterial and venous cerebrovascular disease: preliminary experience. *Radiology* 1994; **191**: 441–446.

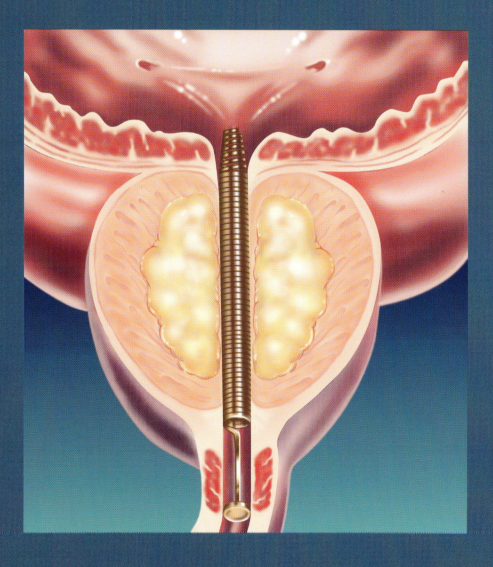

Chapter 11

Metallic stents: individual designs and characteristics

A.F. Watkinson, E.P Strecker and I. Boos

Introduction

A stent is a form of scaffolding that is used to reinforce the patency of a biological conduit by holding the walls apart. It is named after Charles Stent, a British dentist in the late 19th century, who was the inventor of a material used to support skin grafts. The use of scaffolding is not a new concept; indeed, the ancient Egyptians are reported to have used hollow reeds to treat urethral strictures. Modern metallic stents are available in both self-expanding and balloon-expandable designs in a variety of alloys. These include stainless steel, tantalum and nitinol (thermal memory).

Background

As with so many innovations in interventional radiology, it was Charles Dotter in 1969 who first tried polymer tubes in canine peripheral arteries; however, he reported that, regardless of the material from which the stent was made (polyethylene, polyamide or Teflon), no impervious plastic graft remained patent longer than 24 hours. In 6 additional experiments Dotter[1] used metal spirals, 3 uncoated, and 3 coated with silicone. The 3 coated spirals occluded within 24 hours, whereas 2 of the uncoated spirals of length 1 cm remained patent at 2 years follow-up. This early spiral was a very closed design and as a consequence no epithelialization occurred.

Between 1982 and 1984, Maass *et al*. published a series of articles[2–4] reporting their experiences with helical prostheses in the form of monofilaments, in single and double helix format. This group was the first to study in detail the effects of the stent upon the vessel wall. Intimal hyperplasia appeared to be more pronounced in the venous system. Collateral vessels covered by the stent wires remained patent.

In 1982, Hans Wallsten designed a braided cylindrical endoprosthesis that was made in two formats. One was uncovered, and one covered with microporous polyurethane with the objective of sealing aortic aneurysms. The Wallstent endoprosthesis was first used clinically by Rousseau in 1985 when it was implanted into an aortic valve fistula. No anticoagulants were used and it occluded within 6 months.

At about the same time (and shortly afterwards), several stent designs were being developed at a number of independent centres. These included nitinol stents,[5,6] the Gianturco stent,[7] the Palmaz stent[8,9] and the Strecker stent.[10] These have all been subsequently introduced into modern everyday practice in the vascular, biliary, gastrointestinal and urinary systems.

Balloon-expandable stents

These stents are mounted on a Gruntzig-type balloon catheter and are expanded passively by balloon inflation. Once the stents have been expanded by the balloon, and the balloon deflated, they do not expand further. Two types of balloon-expandable stent are commercially available: the Palmaz (Johnson & Johnson Interventional systems, Warren, NJ, USA) and the Strecker (Boston Scientific Inc., Watertown, MA, USA) stents.

Palmaz stent

Palmaz and his colleagues first introduced the concept of the balloon-expandable stent in 1985. The original design involved a tubular meshwork of annealed steel that could be deployed by the use of a coaxial balloon system. After some 300 successful animal implants and up to 3 years of follow-up, the first human Palmaz stent implants, under FDA-approved protocol, were performed in Europe and the United States in 1987. Initially, 24 stents were placed in the iliac arteries of 15 patients. No stent thrombosed or closed abruptly.[11] Since then, many further studies using the Palmaz stent have been completed or are still in progress, with placement of the device in the coronary arteries, the aorta, the renal arteries, the iliac arteries and more recently the infra-iliac arterial tree. The device has also been implanted in the venous system as well as being used for transjugular intrahepatic portosystemic shunting (TIPS).[12]

Stent design characteristics
The Palmaz stent is made of stainless steel: this is a nine-element alloy in the composition of which chromium is a significant contributor. Molybdenum, although present in much smaller quantities, is also important in determining physical performance as well as stabilizing the cystallographic structure.

Surface finishing is also an important consideration. The stent is electropolished at the end of production to produce a chromium-rich surface. The oxidation of this surface to produce chromium oxide prevents further degradation. The polishing process is also designed to produce a positive surface electric potential to reduce thrombogenicity. The manufacturers claim that this charge attracts plasma proteins, thus rendering the stent surface passive prior to the arrival of platelets and white blood cells.

The stent is usually mounted coaxially on an appropriately sized angioplasty balloon by crimping with a special tool (Fig. 11.1a,b). The stent–balloon assembly is preferentially introduced across the lesion to be treated through a guiding catheter; on retraction of this guiding catheter, balloon inflation releases the stent (Fig. 11.1c,d).

The stent is designed such that on full expansion the struts are embedded in the vessel wall in line with the blood flow. Once fully expanded, the struts assume a diamond lattice shape (Fig. 11.1d) and provide a stable framework for

Figure 11.1
The Palmaz balloon-expandable stent. (a) The unexpanded stent. (b) The stent has been mounted on an Olbert balloon (Meadox, Surgimed A/S, DK 3660 Stenlose, Denmark) and crimped tightly with a special tool. (c)Inflation of the balloon expands the stent to the desired diameter. (d) The final expanded stent after deflation and removal of the balloon.

(a)
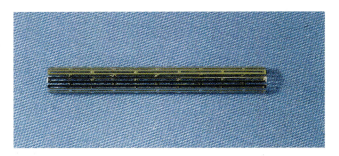

(b)
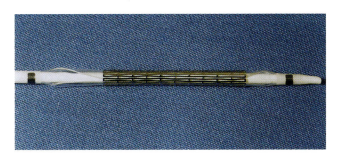

(c)
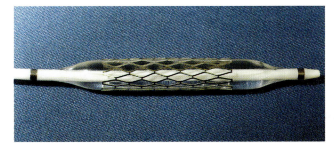

(d)
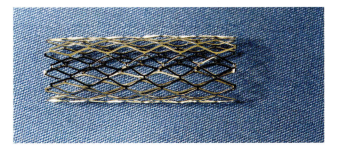

endothelialization to occur. The Palmaz stent has very limited longitudinal flexibility and cannot be applied to very tortuous vessels or used in the crossover technique for a contralateral approach to lower limb vessels. However, the stent can be placed accurately at the desired location, owing to the small amount of shortening that occurs during expansion.

A recent development in the design of the Palmaz stent is the use of heparin coating. The heparin is attached by a covalent bonding process that optimizes activation of the heparinized surface with minimal loss of biochemical effectiveness. The current research work with this prototype device is being performed in the coronary artery; however, this design may have future applications in small vessels with low flow, such as peripheral limb vessels.[13] An articulated stent to increase flexibility is also under investigation.

Strecker stent

In 1987, the first design of the Strecker stent was introduced for clinical use in patients after the completion of animal experiments.[14–16] This was the balloon-expandable vascular tantalum stent, which was first used in iliac and femoral arteries and later in a great variety of arterial sites, as well as in venous lesions and for the treatment of stenosed haemodialysis shunts.

More recently, a knitted self-expanding flexible stent made of nitinol (nickel–titanium compound) was developed for use in other hollow organs, such as the biliary tree, the tracheobronchial tree, the oesophagus and the rectum. In addition, a self-expanding nitinol hexagonal stent has been developed for use in the vascular system and is currently undergoing clinical trials.

Implantation techniques and stent release mechanisms vary with each type of stent and with the organ treated. These are mentioned briefly here and are discussed in more detail in the relevant chapters dealing with the clinical uses of the various stent designs.

Stent design characteristics

The Strecker stent consists of a tubular mesh knitted from a metallic monofilament. The knitting is characterized by loosely connected loops overlapping at their intersections (Fig. 11.2). The stent, which is compressible radially and longitudinally, is mounted on an introduction catheter. With stent release the wire loops widen, with the wire struts moving at their intersections, thus increasing the stent diameter.

The knitted design is flexible, and is compressible in both the radial and longitudinal directions in both the expanded and the non-expanded state. This allows the passage of the catheter–stent assembly through tortuous segments and sharp angulations of any canalicular organ. In addition, the flexibility of the stent is a potential advantage in arterial implantation over articular joints, or other areas where significant movement may take place.

The knitted stent can be retrieved from the implantation site in cases of incorrect placement (Fig. 11.3) with the aid of a special retrieval device[17] (Boston Scientific Inc.).

Percutaneous implantable stents made of tantalum are balloon expandable and used mainly as vascular stents. However, they have also been used in the biliary tree, in the liver for the creation of portosystemic shunts, the tracheobronchial tree and the genitourinary system. The tantalum stent is secured on the balloon by thin-walled silastic sleeves, which are attached to both ends of the balloon and overlap the stent ends by 1–2 mm. The sleeves prevent displacement of the stent from the balloon during advancement through the introducer sheath or passage through curved organs.

Figure 11.2   (a)

The Strecker tantalum stent. (a) The knitted tantalum stent is mounted on the balloon catheter in a compressed fashion and held by silicone sleeves at both ends. (b)With balloon expansion, the stent's wire loops widen with the wire struts moving at their intersections, thus increasing the stent diameter.

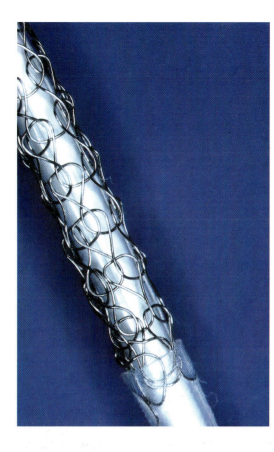

(b)

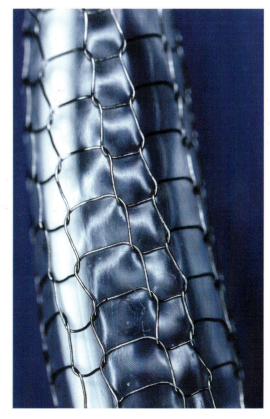

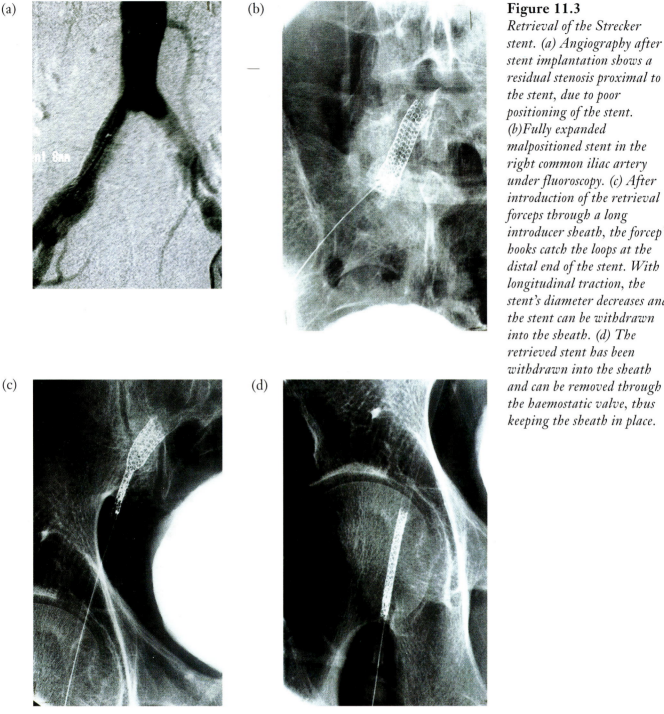

(a)

(b)

(c)

(d)

Figure 11.3
Retrieval of the Strecker stent. (a) Angiography after stent implantation shows a residual stenosis proximal to the stent, due to poor positioning of the stent. (b) Fully expanded malpositioned stent in the right common iliac artery under fluoroscopy. (c) After introduction of the retrieval forceps through a long introducer sheath, the forcep's hooks catch the loops at the distal end of the stent. With longitudinal traction, the stent's diameter decreases and the stent can be withdrawn into the sheath. (d) The retrieved stent has been withdrawn into the sheath and can be removed through the haemostatic valve, thus keeping the sheath in place.

During introduction of the catheter–stent assembly through the haemostatic valve of an introducer sheath, the stent is covered by an additional protection tube to prevent its dislocation from the balloon. After passage of the introducer, the stent is placed at the desired vessel site under fluoroscopic control. Exact stent positioning is facilitated by the tantalum markers of the balloon catheter. The stent is then expanded by balloon inflation. The middle portion of the endoprosthesis expands first, owing to the restraining silastic sleeves at the two ends of the stent. Only when the silastic sleeves retract, on full balloon inflation, are the proximal and distal ends of the stent released (Fig. 11.4). The balloon is removed only after full deflation.

Tantalum has a number of advantages as a stent material due to its metallic properties: because of its radiodensity it is well visualized under fluoroscopy, even when overlaid by dense bone or partially obscured with contrast medium. In addition, tantalum does not interfere with magnetic resonance imaging (MRI) as much as stainless steel,[18–19] because of its non-ferromagnetic properties. This may have important implications in the future both for placement of these devices and in follow-up.

Tantalum is biocompatible and inert, and has been widely used in the surgical field and as an orthopaedic implant material. Studies *in vitro* suggest that tantalum is less thrombogenic than copper, titanium or stainless steel.[20] The thrombogenicity of the stent is further reduced by chemical electropolishing to produce a smooth surface and decrease platelet adhesion. The surface consists of tantalum pentoxide, which is very stable and corrosion resistant.[21–3] In addition, the surface is negatively charged, a characteristic that is claimed by the manufacturers to reduce thrombogenicity by repelling similarly charged platelets.

A nitinol Strecker stent is available for use in the gastrointestinal system, the biliary tree, in the genito-urinary tract, in the creation of portosystemic shunts, and in the tracheobronchial tree. Also a self-expanding *nitinol* hexagonal stent has been developed for use in the vascular system. These stent designs are discussed in the section on nitinol stents.

Self-expanding stents

There are two well-established stainless steel self-expanding endoprostheses: these are the Gianturco–Rösch Z-stent (Cook Inc., Bloomington, IN, USA) and the Wallstent™ endoprosthesis (Schneider AG, Bulach, Switzerland). There are several nitinol self-expanding stents of which the Strecker Elastalloy Ultraflex™

Figure 11.4
Strecker balloon stent assembly. The knitted flexible tantalum stent mounted on a high-pressure 5 Fr balloon catheter. Silicone sleeves secure the stent during insertion, releasing it only as the balloon is inflated. The sleeves roll backwards from the balloon, allowing the centre of the stent to expand fully prior to the ends being released.

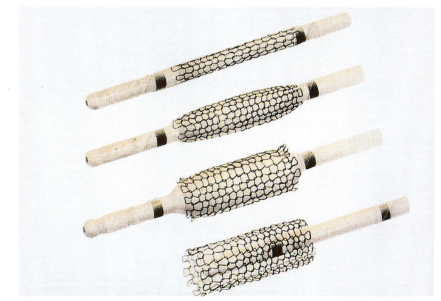

(Boston Scientific Inc.), the Memotherm stent [Angiomed (subsidiary of Bard Inc.) Karlsruhe, Germany] and the Cragg stent (MinTec, Freeport, Grand Bahama, Bahamas) are the most well established. The self-expanding stents have an inherent self-expanding force that contributes towards low stent compressibility following deployment. This minimizes the risk of migration and helps to maintain luminal diameter and therefore patency.

Gianturco Z-stent

In 1985, Gianturco and his associates[7] described an expandable stent made of bare stainless steel wire 0.018 mm in diameter. The wire is bent six to eight times in opposite directions, and the ends joined together to form a cylinder. These zigzag or Z-stents are then compressed to fit in the lumen of a catheter and pushed out of the catheter with a flat-ended pusher (Fig. 11.5a). When the stents extrude beyond the catheter lumen they re-expand to dilate the vessel (Fig. 11.5).

In Gianturco's initial study,[7] Z-stents were placed in the abdominal aorta, the inferior vena cava and the jugular vein of a canine model. Six months after placement there were no flow defects, narrowings or occlusions. The stents were not thrombogenic; no clot formation was observed in any of the stent-containing arteries. Sidebranches that were crossed by stent wires remained patent and there was no stent migration. Within 2–3 weeks of stent placement the stent wires were encased in neointima.

Stent design characteristics

The expansile capability of the stents was determined by the diameter of the wire used, the angle of the bends and the number of the bends. Compared with other designs the stents were fairly rigid and unsuitable for use in small, tortuous arteries. Gianturco originally used the bare Z-stents to relieve obstructions of the superior and inferior vena cava. When he discovered that single Z-stents were frequently misplaced, because of the difficulty of positioning the central portion of the stent precisely over a short stricture, Gianturco built double stents to minimize this problem. He also found that some resistant stenoses/occlusions could not be completely opened with a double stent; however, additional single stents placed inside the initial stent at the junction of the two segments of the double stent – its weakest point – increased the radial expanding force, leading to full expansion.

Various modifications of the stent were introduced to increase flexibility and prevent tumour ingrowth. Uchida and Rösch passed suture material through eyelets made at the bends to increase flexibility. Rösch covered the bare stents with silicone material, while Wright and Gianturco covered them with siliconized Dacron fabric. Both of these techniques temporarily reduced tumour ingrowth through the stent struts.

Shortly before his death in 1985, Andreas Grüntzig asked Gianturco to design and build a stent for use in the coronary arteries in an attempt to address the problem of restenosis. The stent needed to be small to negotiate the tortuosity of the coronary arteries. Gianturco and Roubin eventually designed a balloon-expandable stent for use in the coronary arteries that has subsequently been implanted in over 800 patients.

In 1986,[24] Charnsangavej reported the use of Gianturco stents in the relief of malignant obstruction of the superior and inferior vena cava in two separate

Figure 11.5
The Gianturco Z-stent. (a) The zigzag or Z-stent has been compressed to fit in the lumen of a catheter. When pushed out of the catheter with a flat-ended pusher the stent re-expands to dilate the vessel. (b) The stents are available in a variety of lengths by adding on adjoining sections.

(a)

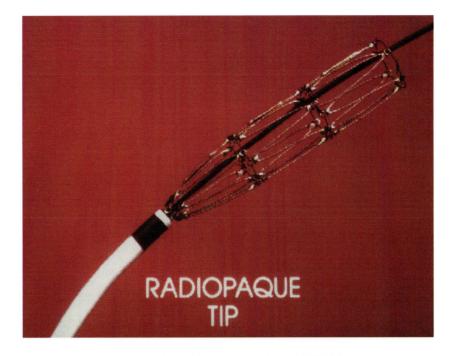

(b)

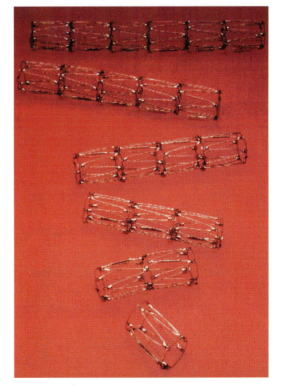

cases. Multiple stents were used in both patients with good palliation of symptoms, although one stent migrated into the right ventricle with no clinical sequelae.

In 1987,[25] Rollins reported that Gianturco Z-stents were effective in atherosclerotic animal models. Eighteen stents were placed in 6 rabbit aortas and left *in situ* for 8 weeks. The ratio of stented to unstented diameters was 1.2:1.

Where the stents were in contact with the vessel wall they became encased in neointima, but the areas of the stents that bridged side vessels were free of intima, thrombus and fibrin. According to this report, the effects of vessel dilatation with expandable stents differ from those of balloon dilatation: the latter is more likely to split the plaque, whereas self-expanding stents dilate the vessel by stretching and compressing the intima and media. Histological examination of the rabbit aortas indicated that the tissue response to Gianturco stents (which exert a continuous, dynamic self-expansile force) differed from the tissue response to angioplasty and placement of a passive endoprosthesis.

Having successfully re-established and maintained patency in occluded large vessels, Duprat et al.[26] in 1987 turned their attention to the possibility of stenting small vessels to maintain patency following angioplasty. Thirty-three expandable metallic Gianturco stents, 3, 4 and 5 mm in diameter (when fully expanded) were placed in small vessels in a canine model. No anticoagulants were given. The success rate was 100% with stents 4 and 5 mm in diameter and 54% with 3 mm stents. None of the stents migrated or perforated the vessel wall. All side vessels bridged by the stents were patent and had not become narrowed. The relationship of stent diameter to lumen diameter, termed the stent-to-artery ratio (SAR), was crucial. When the SAR exceeded 1.2, complications occurred, including thrombosis with or without recanalization, vessel spasm, and excessive intimal proliferation over the stent wires. An SAR of 1.2 or less, however, resulted in an angiographic success rate of 100%.

Gianturco Z-stents are now available for biliary, venous and tracheobrochial applications, and a covered version has been developed for oesophageal use. The Gianturco Roubin Flex Coronary stent is now in its second generation.

The Wallstent endoprosthesis

The self-expanding metallic Wallstent endoprosthesis was first patented in 1982 by Hans Wallsten, then President of Medinvent SA, a research and design company based in Lausanne, Switzerland. This original Wallstent endoprosthesis was of a braided, cylindrical design and was produced in two formats for animal work — uncovered to treat stenoses and occlusions, and a version covered with microporous polyurethane with the objective of sealing aortic aneurysms.

The uncovered Wallstent was first used clinically in Toulouse by Rousseau, when it was implanted in a haemodialysis arteriovenous fistula. No anticoagulation was given and the stent occluded within 6 months. In 1986, Puel carried out the first implantation of a Wallstent endoprosthesis into a coronary artery; the stent remained patent.

In 1989, Medinvent SA was purchased by Schneider International and research and production moved to Zurich. Since that time development has been rapid, with stents currently available for use in the vascular system,[27–9] the biliary system,[30–32] the oesophagus,[33] the tracheo-bronchial tree[34] and as a stent for portosystemic shunts.[35] New developments include the design of a covered stent to prevent tumour ingrowth and to seal fistulae (Fig. 11.6), stents with increased radio-opacity and the design of new delivery systems. In the initial design of the covered oesophageal stent the polyurethane covering was outside the metallic filaments; this predisposed the stent to migration, especially when the lower end of the endoprosthesis projected into the fundus of the stomach. In a new design, currently undergoing clinical trials, the polyurethane covering is inside the

Figure 11.6
The uncovered 22 mm (top) and polyurethane-covered 25 mm oesophageal Wallstents.

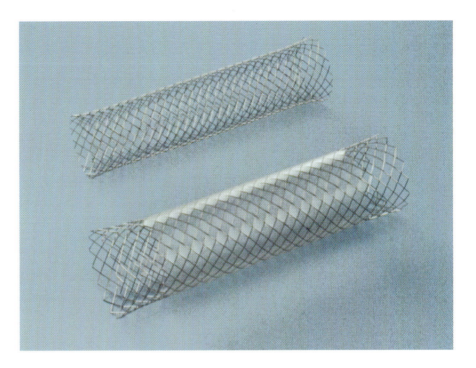

metallic filaments. This increases friction between the stent and the wall of the oesophagus, reducing the risk of migration (A. Adam, personal communication).

Stent design characteristics
This is a self-expanding stent that has a cylindrical braided structure (Fig. 11.7) composed of 24 wires of 0.12 mm diameter in the vascular and biliary endoprostheses (this varies for the coronary stent). Variations in stent design include the use of a cobalt-based alloy with six tungsten wires for improved radio-

Figure 11.7
The Wallstent endoprosthesis. The flexibility of the stent is ideally suited to tortuous vessels and placement via a contralateral approach.

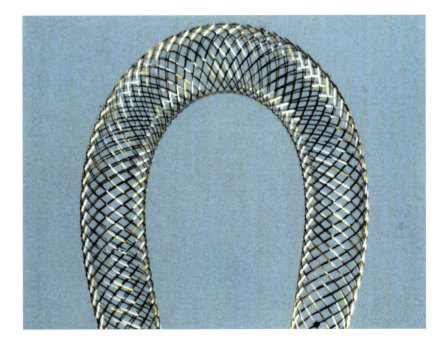

opacity, and drawn filled tubing. In this latter design (for vascular use), each wire of the stent has a core of either tantalum or platinum for improved radio-opacity and a jacket of cobalt-based alloy.

The stent has an intrinsic expansile force and no fixed cross-points, a design that allows it to conform to the shape of the vessel with longitudinal and axial flexibility. The stent is elongated, to allow it to be mounted on to a delivery system of small diameter, and shortens and expands on release. The degree of shortening is dependent upon the diameter to which the Wallstent expands, and also the mesh angle: the narrower the mesh angle the less shortening will occur (Fig. 11.8). This mesh angle also affects the strength of the radial force, which becomes smaller as the angle narrows. The Wallstent has two mesh angles (> 140 degrees and < 120 degrees) (Fig. 11.8).

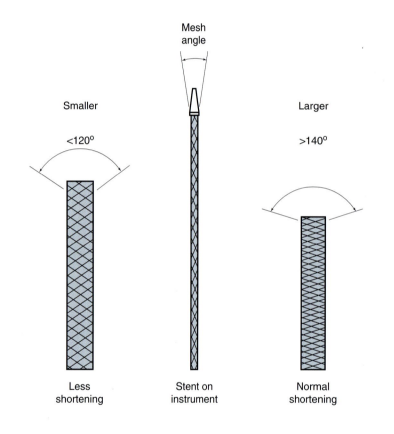

Figure 11.8
The influence of the mesh angle of the Wallstent endoprosthesis on expansile force and shortening.

Delivery systems
The rolling membrane system (Fig. 11.9). This is the original stent release design, which allows progressive controlled release while enabling proximal repositioning prior to full release. The delivery system is available in sizes of 5 (coronary circulation), 7 and 9 Fr. The 7 and 9 Fr delivery catheters are tapered to a guidewire of maximum 0.038 inch; the 5 Fr delivery catheter is tapered to a 0.018 inch guidewire. The flexibility of the system allows implantation of the Wallstent in the contralateral iliac artery using the crossover technique. The Wallstent is elongated and mounted near the tip of the delivery catheter; it is secured to the catheter by a double invaginated polyurethane membrane. To release the

Figure 11.9
The rolling membrane Wallstent delivery system. (a) The unreleased stent. (b) Partial release of the stent by withdrawal of the outer constraining membrane. (c) Full release of the stent. Note how the stent has shortened with expansion.

(a)

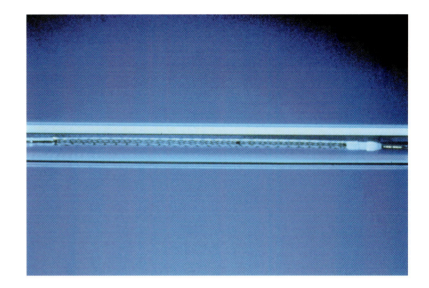

(b)

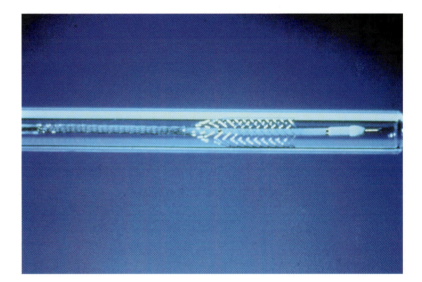

(c)

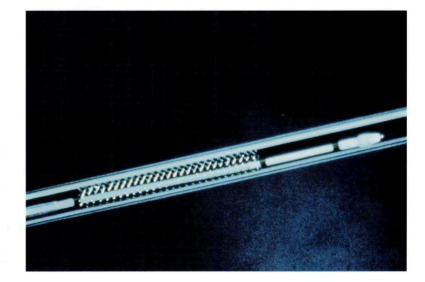

Wallstent, contrast medium is infused, under pressure, into the space between the membranes, causing them to separate. The membrane can then be gradually retracted, allowing the stent to expand owing to the intrinsic radial expansile force. Prior to release, proximal repositioning is possible after reapplication of the vacuum between the two layers of the rolling membrane (this is necessary to prevent inadvertent release during repositioning).

Telestep delivery system. The covered Wallstent (for use in the oesophagus and respiratory tree) is mounted on this delivery system and is available in 15, 18 and 22 Fr sizes. The stent is released by withdrawal of an outer sheath, which releases the distal 50% of the stent. If repositioning is required, advancement of this outer sheath, at this point, will enable the stent to be recovered. To release the stent fully, after withdrawal of the outer sheath, a middle sheath is pulled back to complete the release. If more than 50% of the stent has been released, then repositioning of the stent is not possible.

Rigistep delivery system. This delivery system has been developed for the tracheobronchial Wallstent to facilitate implantation under direct visual control during bronchoscopy and integrated venturi jet ventilation. The delivery system is reusable and of similar design to a rigid bronchoscope, allowing mounting of a stent of appropriate size at the time of the procedure. The stent is released by withdrawing the outer steel tube to reveal the endoprosthesis. No repositioning is possible during release.

Placehit Wallstent delivery system (Fig. 11.10). This delivery system, which is intended eventually to replace the rolling membrane system, has been developed to facilitate ease of introduction, and to allow proximal and distal repositioning during stent release. Currently, this system is available for transhepatic use in the biliary tree, for insertion of uncovered oesophageal stents and for venous use in the vena cava. The stent is released by withdrawing the covering sheath. If the

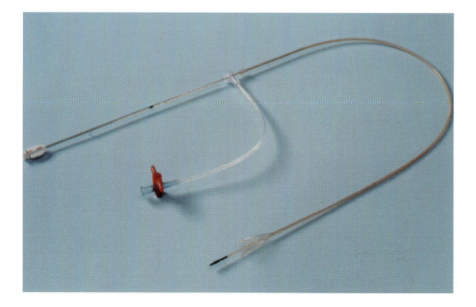

Figure 11.10
The Placehit Wallstent delivery system.

outer sheath is withdrawn to the repositioning marker on the inner steel tube, then 50% of the stent has been released. Recovering and proximal or distal repositioning is possible until this point; beyond this marker, this manoeuvre should not be attempted.

Nitinol stents

Nitinol is a binary compound of nickel and titanium that expands and contracts owing to the effect of temperature. Its superelastic properties are based on a 'shape memory effect' that is gained by heat treatment of the raw material. The nitinol stent, therefore, tends always to regain its preset shape and size and thus behaves as a self-expanding stent. Nitinol is non-thrombogenic, biocompatible and non-paramagnetic. During manufacture of the nitinol alloy, any excursion outside tolerance levels of 1 part in 10,000 will render the alloy useless for manufacture of thermoreactive stents.

Apart from its superelastic qualities, nitinol is known for its resistance to sustained strain, excellent biocompatibility and corrosion resistance.[36-9] No corrosion has been observed in clinical experiments either macroscopically[40] or with histomorphological evaluation.[41]

The feature of shape memory of nitinol for stent design was first applied by Dotter[5] and Cragg[6] in animal experiments. More recently, Rabkin[42-3] renewed efforts to use nitinol stents for both vascular and non-vascular applications.

Currently, the three most commonly used self-expanding nitinol stents are the Strecker Elastalloy Ultraflex (TM)(Boston Scientific Inc., Watertown, MA, USA), the Memotherm stent (Angiomed [subsidiary of Bard Inc.] Karlsruhe, Germany) and the Cragg stent (MinTec, Freeport, Grand Bahama, Bahamas).

Strecker Elastalloy Ultraflex (Fig. 11.11).

This prosthesis has been used widely in the gastrointestinal tract; more recently, stents have become available for use in the biliary tree, for the creation of portosystemic shunts and in the tracheobronchial tree. The stent is knitted from highly elastic nitinol wire of varying diameter (biliary 0.13 mm, oesophageal 0.15 mm) and is flexible in both radial and longitudinal directions. The larger oesophageal and rectal stents are stretched and compressed in a low-profile manner and embedded in gelatin. On withdrawal of an outer sheath, the gelatin comes into contact with body fluids and dissolves to release the stent. A new covered Strecker oesophageal stent has recently been developed to counter the problem of tumour ingrowth and to enable sealing of oesophageal fistulae.

The biliary and genitourinary tract nitinol stents are loaded onto a 10 Fr sheath and are self-expanding on withdrawal of an outer sheath. The stent shortens approximately 35% on release and correct positioning is aided by radio-opaque markers demonstrating the position of the restrained and fully expanded stent.

The tracheobronchial superelastic nitinol Strecker stent is mounted on an introducer catheter and is released by a special release mechanism involving a restraining textile mesh.[44] A similar release mechanism is used in the new covered oesophageal Strecker stent. Retraction of a retaining thread unravels the encircling mesh, thus releasing the stent.

(a)

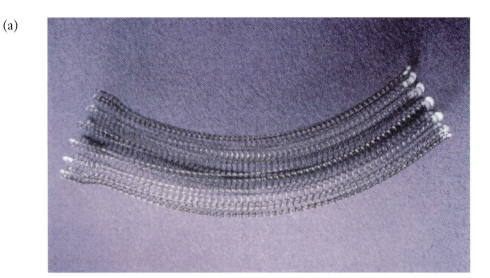

Figure 11.11
The Strecker Elastalloy Ultraflex. (a) The unconstrained 10 cm long, 18 mm diameter oesophageal endoprosthesis. (b) and (c) Magnified views of the flared tip, demonstrating the interlocking woven nitinol wire. This allows both longitudinal and radial flexibility.

(b)

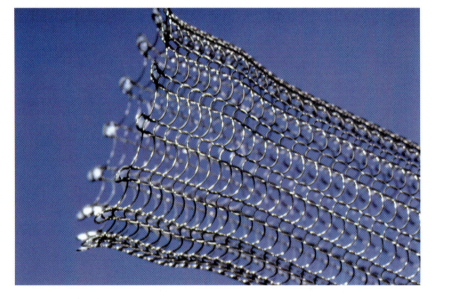

(c)

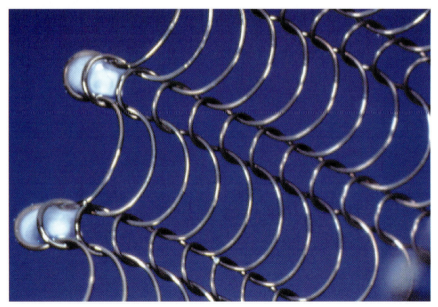

Memotherm (Angiomed) nitinol stent (Fig. 11.12)

The Memotherm stent was designed and manufactured by Angiomed in Karlsruhe, Germany and was released for general use in 1993. It is a self-expanding, single-walled nitinol stent that is thermoreactive. The particular blend of nitinol used to manufacture the Memotherm stent attains maximum expansion (and hence maximum predetermined diameter and radial force) at 35.5°C. Above this temperature it attains no further expansion or increased radial force.

During manufacture the stent mesh is laser-cut from a single tube of nitinol. The aim of this process is to ensure that no welds or joins in the stent surface are present, in order to provide a smooth stent surface and minimize turbulence. The stent is shaped over a forming mandrel that determines the exact length and diameter. This preformed stent then undergoes 16 successive heat treatments to modify the crystal structure and give it its thermal memory. The stent ends are slightly flared to minimize the risk of migration (Fig. 11.12). As a final process, the internal surface is polished to reduce thrombogenicity and turbulence. In addition, the stent carries a negative surface electrostatic charge to limit platelet adhesion and further reduce the risk of thrombus formation.

The introduction system comprises a coaxial catheter sheath system that tracks over a standard 0.035 in guidewire (Fig. 11.13). The stent comes premounted on the inner of the two catheters, the outer catheter covering the stent; it is inserted via an introducer sheath. There are two highly opaque platinum markers, the proximal one on the inner catheter and the distal marker on the outer catheter, relating to the proximal and distal extent of the stent after deployment. The coaxial catheter system is attached to a pistol grip (Fig. 11.13a). The stent is deployed by pulling the trigger of the pistol grip, after first removing the safety catch. Each pull of the trigger pulls the outer catheter back 0.5 cm. As the outer catheter moves back, the stent reaches body temperature and expands. To ensure accurate deployment it is best to exert a slight back pressure on the pistol; this ensures that the stent does not move forward during placement. Care must also be taken to ensure that the proximal marker remains still during deployment. The distal marker moves back towards the pistol as the outer sheath moves back and the stent deploys. Minor repositioning is possible as long as the stent is not fully

Figure 11.12
The Angiomed Memotherm nitinol stent.

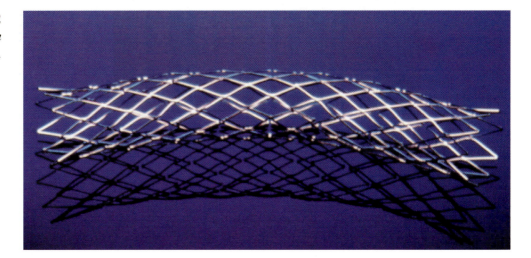

(a)

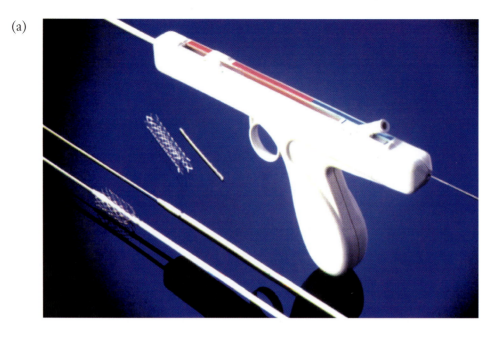

Figure 11.13
The Angiomed Memotherm nitinol stent. (a) The coaxial catheter sheath system attached to a pistol grip. (b) Magnified view of the tip of the sheath system after partial release of the stent.

(b)

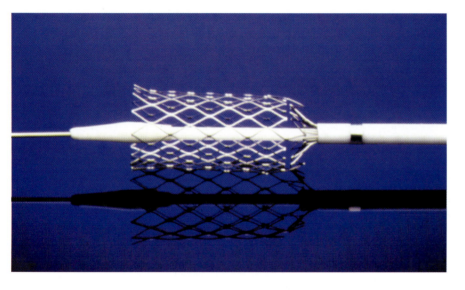

anchored. For an iliac stent, this would be after approximately 5% of the stent had been released. The stent undergoes only minimal foreshortening (less than 3%): the constrained and released lengths are therefore approximately the same; this contributes to accurate, controlled stent placement. Another advantage of the Memotherm stent is its high radio-opacity, which makes it easily visible on fluoroscopy.

Even though the stent was not introduced until 1993, it has found wide application and currently devices are available for use in the arterial, venous, biliary and renal systems. In addition, a TIPS and TIPS reduction stent are obtainable. As the Memotherm stent has been in use for a relatively short period, data are only now becoming available on the performance in these various applications.[45–7]

Future developments are aimed towards endoscopically placed biliary stents, covered and uncovered oesophageal stents, coronary stents and a covered stent system for the treatment of abdominal aortic aneurysms.

Cragg stent, Cragg Endopro and the Stentor aortic graft stent (Mintec Ltd)

These devices are made of nitinol. Uncovered and covered (ultrathin prosthetic graft) Cragg stents have been used in the vascular system with particular application in occlusive and aneurysmal disease. Most experience has been obtained in the iliac and femoral arteries,[48–51] with good initial results.

The *uncovered Cragg stent* (Fig. 11.14) is constructed by winding a monofilament of 0.028 cm nitinol wire on a metal mandrel. The wire is wound on the mandrel such that a series of back-and-forth bends is created in a spiral fashion around the circumference of the mandrel. The distance between the bends is 4 mm. When completed, the wire configuration consists of a tubular shape of longitudinally orientated back-and-forth bends.

Annealing the stent prior to removal from the mandrel imparts it with a thermal memory. Finally, the apices of each abutting loop are fixed with a single ligature of 7/0 polypropylene suture. This increases the hoop strength of the

Figure 11.14
The uncovered nitinol Cragg stent. (a) Magnified view of the stent after partial release from the introducing Teflon capsule. The restraining polypropylene sutures are clearly visible. (b) The fully released stent demonstrating good flexibility.

(a)

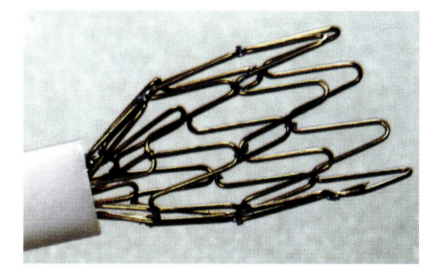

(b)

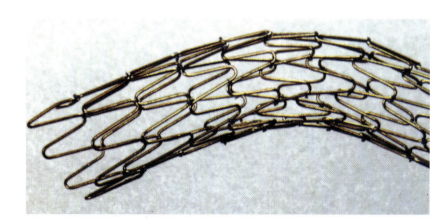

stent; in laboratory studies the hoop strength was greater than that of the Wallstent on compression testing,[48] but the endoprosthesis still maintained good longitudinal flexibility. Suturing of the abutting loops also facilitates introduction.

The stent comes preloaded in an 8.5 Fr Teflon capsule with a constrained diameter of 2.5 mm. At body temperature the stent expands to a predetermined diameter of 8 or 10 mm and shortens by approximately 7%. An 8.5 Fr 30 cm introducer sheath is positioned across the occluded iliac segment and the preloaded stent is inserted into the sheath from the loading capsule. A blunt positioning catheter allows positioning of the stent under fluoroscopic guidance. Withdrawal of the sheath while maintaining the blunt catheter position will release the stent (Fig. 11.14a). Positioning is facilitated by radio-opaque proximal and distal platinum markers. Introduction of the stent is aided by slow infusion of cold saline into the Teflon loading capsule and also during introduction through the introducer sheath. This keeps the wire in the softened constrained state.

The *covered Cragg Endopro* is a Cragg nitinol stent covered with a woven fabric graft (Fig. 11.15). As previously noted, if the stent is cooled in cold saline, the material becomes soft and can be deformed without losing the memory of shape. When warmed to a transition temperature, the wire resumes its original annealed shape. The stent cover is a prosthetic graft of ultrathin (0.1 mm thick), low-porosity woven Dacron, which is coated with a low-molecular-weight heparin. The Dacron is attached to the nitinol stent with the same ligatures of 7/0 polypropylene that are used to stabilize the zigzag loops.

A 9 Fr 50 cm long introducer sheath is used and positioned across the diseased iliac segment, whether occlusive or aneurysmal. The delivery system is very similar to that of the uncovered design, with the graft preloaded in a Teflon cartridge. The graft can then be transferred to the introducer sheath, using a blunt positioning catheter, and advanced across the diseased segment under fluoroscopic guidance. Withdrawal of the sheath while maintaining the blunt catheter position will release the stent. Positioning is again facilitated by radio-opaque proximal and distal platinum markers. Introduction of a slowly infusing cold saline solution will again keep the stent in a soft constrained state until deployment.

Progress in interventional radiology has made it possible to treat abdominal aortic aneurysms (AAA) using self-expanding, metallic stents covered with a low-permeability, polyester fabric.[52] At the present time there is no commercially available endovascular device that is specifically designed to treat AAA, although several such designs are currently being tested, of which the Stentor device is one.

The *Stentor aortic graft stent* is an enlarged version of the Cragg Endopro system. It is a flexible self-expanding endoprosthesis constructed from the same nitinol monofilament wire and sutured together with 7/0 polypropylene ligatures. This basic stent design is covered with a low-permeability polyester fabric. There are two basic designs — a bifurcated (STB) and a straight tube (STS). The proximal and distal ends are tagged by a platinum marker to assist in positioning. The STB consists of two pieces that are introduced from separate groins and mated *in vivo*: these are (1) the aortic section with a single limb and (2) the second limb. At the distal part of the aortic section (STB) there is a short branch (stump) into which the second contralateral iliac limb is inserted. The junction where the two sections are connected is tagged by platinum markers to aid in their mating. The STB is introduced through an 18 Fr delivery catheter with a balloon on the

Figure 11.15
The covered Cragg Endopro. (a) Magnified view from the end of the stent, showing the outer woven Dacron coating and the inner nitinol supporting stent with restraining polypropylene sutures. (b) The stent from the inside. The structure of the low-porosity Dacron can now be seen.

(a)

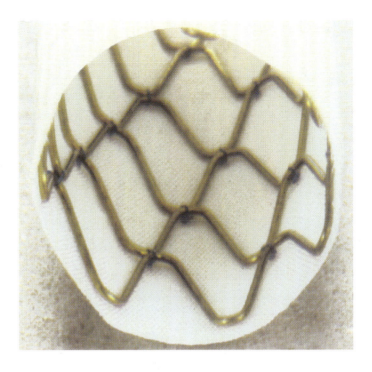

(b)

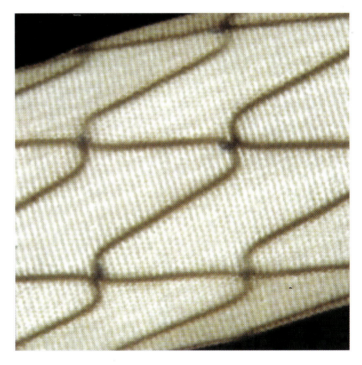

distal end to allow aortic obstruction above the renal arteries and subsequent remodelling of the proximal section of the stent frame into the aortic neck.

Further stent designs relevant to treatment of AAA have been discussed in previous chapters.

In addition to the Elastalloy nitinol stent, Boston Scientific have recently developed a new self-expanding nitinol vascular stent. This is formed of a single strand of nickel–titanium alloy configured to form a tubular implant of hexagonal cell patterns (Fig. 11.16). It is a thermal memory stent designed to expand to a predetermined diameter at body temperature. It is preloaded into a catheter in its unexpanded state and is restrained by an outer sleeve. The restraining sheath is positioned across the implant site and retracted against an internal pusher to release the stent. It has been designed to encompass the attributes of a self-expanding stent (flexibility, longer available lengths and resistance to external compression) and maintain accuracy of placement, as there is very little foreshortening on release. The stent is currently undergoing final clinical trials and at the time of going to press is not yet widely available.

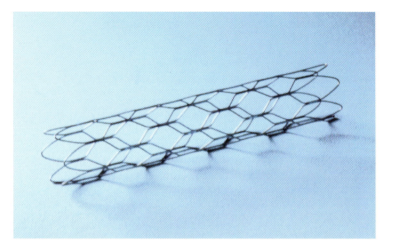

Figure 11.16
The self-expanding nitinol hexagonal vascular stent.

New developments

Since percutaneous implantable stents have been introduced for the treatment of peripheral artery occlusive disease, these new devices have opened the field for a variety of interventional treatment modalities. Today, stent therapy is widely accepted for interventional treatment in the vascular as well as in the non-vascular area. With experience, new indications have been added, rendering possible percutaneous treatment of lesions that were formerly submitted to surgery. The use of tubular and bifurcated aortic stents and low-profile intravascular bypass grafts is currently being evaluated. The long-term success of stent therapy is diminished by restenosis, whether this be due to intimal hyperplasia or tumour ingrowth. The application of endovascular stents, especially in small-diameter arteries, is impaired mainly by restenosis due to myointimal proliferation, which, so far, cannot be reduced by any systemically applied medical therapy. Current research in stent design, as well as concentrating on improved stent technology, includes covered stents, coated stents and drug-releasing stents. The use of a polylactide covering membrane that is biocompatible and biodegradable, resulting in elution of an incorporated drug, has been investigated on tantalum arterial stents.[53] Early results from the use of angiogenesis inhibitor-coated metallic stents in porcine bile ducts shows promise in preventing benign reactive overgrowth.[54]

In addition, the use of pre- and post-stent implantation radiation therapy[55-6] may limit neointima formation and contribute to improved long-term stent patency. High-frequency induction heating of stents is also under investigation to reduce intimal hyperplasia and control tumour ingrowth.[57]

In conclusion, the recent interest in the use of metallic endoprostheses has contributed significantly to patient management in a wide variety of disease processes. The constant revision and refinement of stent designs will continue to attempt to overcome the problems of stent occlusion due to thrombus, intimal hyperplasia or tumour ingrowth.

References

1   Dotter CT. Transluminally placed coilspring endarterectomy tube grafts: long-term patency in canine popliteal artery. *Invest Radiol* 1969; **4**: 327–332.

2   Maass D, Kropf L, Egloff L *et al*. Transluminal implantation of intravascular 'double helix' spiral prostheses: technical and biological considerations. *ESAO Proc* 1982; **9**: 252–256.

3   Maass D, Demierre D, Deaton D *et al*. Transluminal implantation of self-adjusting expandable prostheses: principles, techniques and results. *Prog Artif Org* 1983; 979–987.

4   Maass D, Zollikofer CHL, Largiader F *et al*. Radiological follow-up of transluminally inserted vascular endoprostheses: an experimental study using expanding spirals. *Radiology* 1984; **152**: 659–663.

5   Dotter CT, Buschmann RW, McKinney MK *et al*. Transluminally expandable nitinol coil stent grafting: preliminary results. *Radiology* 1983; **147**: 259–260.

6   Cragg A, Lund G, Rysavy J *et al*. Nonsurgical placement of arterial endoprostheses: a new technique using nitinol wire. *Radiology* 1983; **147**: 261–263.

7   Wright KC, Wallace S, Charnsangavej C *et al*. Percutaneous endovascular stents: an experimental evaluation. *Radiology* 1985; **156**: 69–72.

8   Palmaz JC, Sibbitt RR, Reuter STR *et al*. Expandable intraluminal graft: a preliminary study. *Radiology* 1985; **156**: 73–77.

9   Palmaz JC, Windeler SA, Gaarcia F *et al*. Atherosclerotic rabbit aortas: expandable intraluminal grafting. *Radiology* 1986; **160**: 723–726.

10 Strecker EP, Berg C, Weber H *et al* Experimentelle Untersuchung mit einer neuen perkutan einfuhrbaren und aufdehnbaren Gefassendoprothese. *Fortschr Rontgenstr* 1987; **147**: 669–672.

11 Palmaz JC, Schatz RA, Richter G *et al*. Intraluminal stenting of iliac artery stenosis: preliminary report of a multi centre study. *Circulation* 1988; **78**(Suppl. III): 415.

12 Richter GM, Palmaz JC, Noeldge G *et al*. Der transjugulare intrahepatische portosystemische Stent-Shunt (TIPSS). *Radiologe* 1989; **29**: 406–411.

13 Serruys P. Benestent II pilot results. AHA meeting abstract. 1995.

14 Strecker EP, Romaniuk P, Schneider B *et al*. Perkutan implantierbare, durch Ballon aufdehnbare GefaBprothese: Erste klinische Ergebnisse. *Dtsch Med Wochenschr* 1988; **113**: 538.

15 Strecker EP, Liermann D, Barth KH *et al*. Expandable tubular stents for treatment of arterial occlusive disease: experimental and clinical results. *Radiology* 1990; **175**: 97.

16 Barth KH, Virmaani R, Strecker EP *et al*. Flexible tantalum stents implanted in aortas and iliac arteries: effect in normal canines. *Radiology* 1990; **175**: 91–96.

17 Liermann D. Temporary stenting. In: Liermann D (ed.) *Stents – State of the art and future developments*. Morin Heights, Canada: Polyscience Publications Inc., 1995; in conjunction with Boston Scientific Corporation, Watertown, MA. USA: 329–338.

18 Matsumoto AH, Teitelbaum GP, Barth KH *et al*. Tantalum vascular stents: in vivo evaluation with MR imaging. *Radiology* 1989; **170**: 753–755.

19 Laissy JP, Grand C, Matos C *et al*. Magnetic Resonance angiography of intravascular endoprostheses : investigation of three devices. *Cardiovasc Intervent Radiol* 1995; **18**: 360–366.

20 Hearn JA, Robinson KA, Roubin. In vitro thrombus formation of stent wires: role of metallic composition and heparin coating (abstract). *J Am Coll Cardiol* 1991; **17**: 302A.

21 Zitter H, Plenk H. The electrochemical behaviour of metallic implant materials as an indicator of their biocompatibility. *J Biomed Mater Res* 1987; **21**: 881–896.

22 von Holst H, Collins P, Steiner L. Titanium, silver and tantalum clips in brain tissue. *Acta Neurochir* 1981; **56**: 239–242.

23 Bomas L, Laurent A, Sapoval M. Accelerated stent ageing: study by electrocorrosion. In: Liermann D (ed.) *Stents – State of the art and future developments*. Morin Heights, Canada: Polyscience Publications Inc. 1995; in conjunction with Boston Scientific Corporation, Watertown, MA, USA: 279–283.

24 Charnsangavej C, Carrasco H, Wallace S *et al*. Stenosis of the vena cava: preliminary assessment of treatment with expandable metal stents. *Radiology* 1986; **161**: 295–298.

25 Rollins N, Wright KC, Charnsangavej C *et al*. Self-expanding metallic stents: preliminary evaluation in an atherosclerotic model. *Radiology* 1987; **163**: 739–742.

26 Duprat G, Wright KC, Charnsangavej C *et al*. Flexible balloon-expanded stent for small vessels. *Radiology* 1987; **162**: 276–278.

27 Sigwart V, Puel J, Mirkovitch V *et al*. Intravascular stents to prevent occlusion and restenosis after transluminal angioplasty. *N Engl J Med* 1987; **316**: 701–706.

28 Zollikofer CHL, Largiader I, Bruhlmann WF *et al*. Endovascular stenting of veins and grafts: preliminary experience. *Radiology* 1988; **167**: 707–712.

29 Watkinson AF, Hansell DM, Expandable Wallstent for the treatment of obstruction of the superior vena cava. *Thorax* 1993; **48**: 915–920.

30 Gillams A, Dick R, Dooley JS *et al*. Self-expandable stainless steel braided endoprosthesis for biliary strictures. *Radiology* 1990; **174**: 137–140.

31 Adam A, Chetty N, Roddie M *et al*. Self-expandable stainless steel endoprostheses for treatment of malignant bile duct obstruction. *AJR* 1991; **156**: 321–325.

32 Lameris JS, Stoker J, Nijs HGT *et al*. Malignant biliary obstruction: percutaneous use of self-expandable stents. *Radiology* 1991; **179**: 703–707.

33 Watkinson AF, Ellul J, Entwisle K *et al*. Esophageal carcinoma: initial results of palliative treatment with covered self-expanding endoprostheses. *Radiology* 1995; **195**: 821–827.

34 Rousseau H, Dahan M, Lauque D *et al*. Self-expanding endoprostheses in the tracheobronchial tree. *Radiology* 1993; **188**: 199–203.

35 LaBerge JM, Ring EJ, Gordon RL *et al*. Creation of transjugular intrahepatic portosystemic shunts with the Wallstent endoprosthesis: results in 100 patients. *Radiology* 1993; **187**: 413–420.

36 Buhler WJ, Wang FE. A summary of recent research in the nitinol alloys and their potential applications in ocean engineering. *Ocean Eng* 1968; **1**: 105–120.

37 Tietze H. Phasenubergange mit Memory-Effekt. Frankfurt: Verlag f. akademische Schriften, 1985.

38 Lucas L, Dale P, Buchanan R *et al*. In vitro and in vivo corrosion analyses of implant alloys. 2nd world congress on biomaterials, 10th annual meeting of the Society for Biomaterials, Washington, DC, USA: 27 April–1 May 1984: 182.

39 Oonishi H, Tsuji E, Miyaga N *et al*. In vitro and in vivo corrosion analyses of implant alloys. 2nd world congress on biomaterials, 10th annual meeting of the Society for Biomaterials, Washington, DC, USA: 27 April–1 May 1984: 183.

40 Edie JW, Andreasen GF, Zaytoun MP. Surface corrosion of nitinol and stainless steel under clinical conditions. *Angle Orthod* 1981; **51**: 319–324.

41 Grewe P, Krampe K, Muller KM *et al*. Macroscopic and histopathologic alterations of the bronchial wall after implantation of nitinol stents. In: Liermann D (ed.) *Stents – State of the art and future developments*. Morin Heights, Canada: Polyscience Publications Inc., 1995; in conjunction with Boston Scientific Corporation, Watertown, MA, USA: 256–259.

42 Rabkin JK. New types of technology in roentgenosurgery. IX. All-unions Konress uber Frotschritte in der Roentgen-Chirurgie. Moskau, USSR 1989.

43 Rabkin JK, Natzvlishvili ZG, Kavtelladze ZA. Seven years experience with Rabkin technology nitinol endoprostheses for vessels after balloon, laser and rotor recanalisation. National Research Centre of Surgery. Moscow, USSR 1991.

44 Becker HD, Wagner B, Liermann D *et al*. Stenting of the central airways. In: Liermann D (ed.) *Stents – State of the art and future developments*. Morin Heights, Canada: Polyscience Publications Inc. 1995; in conjunction with Boston Scientific Corporation, Watertown, MA, USA: 249–255.

45 Hauenstein KH, Haag K, Ochs A *et al*. The reducing stent: treatment for transjugular intrahepatic portosystemic shunt-induced refractory hepatic encephalopathy and liver failure. *Radiology* 1995; **194**: 175–179.

46 Stark EE, Dukiet C, Truss J *et al*. Strecker-Tantalum and Memotherm-Nitinol stents: comparison of clinical data. *Radiology* 1995; **197**: 1160(P), 316.

47 Friedrich JM, Vogel J, Goerich J. Usefulness of a new Nitinol stent in treatment of biliary obstructions. *Radiology* 1995; **197**: 696(P), 241.

48 Cragg AH, De Jong SC, Barnhart WH *et al*. Nitinol intravascular stent: results of preclinical evaluation. *Radiology* 1993; **189**: 775–778.

49 Henry M, Amor M, Ethevenot G *et al*. Initial experience with the Cragg Endopro system 1 for intraluminal treatment of peripheral vascular disease. *J Endovasc Surg* 1994; **1**: 31–33.

50 Hausegger KA, Cragg AH, Lammer J *et al*. Iliac artery stent placement: clinical experience with a nitinol stent. *Radiology* 1994; **190**: 199–202.

51 Pernes JM, Auguste MA, Hovasse D *et al*. Long iliac stenosis: initial clinical experience with the Cragg endoluminal graft. *Radiology* 1995; **196**: 67–71.

52 Parodi JC, Palmaz JC, Barone HD. Traitement des aneurysmes de l'aorte abdominale par prothèse endoluminale mise en place par voie femorale. *Ann Chir Vasc* 1991; **5**: 491–499.

53 Strecker EP, Hagen B, Liermann D *et al*. Current status of the Strecker stent. *Cardiol Clin* 1994; **12**: 673–687.

54 Machan LS, Jessurun MD, Hunter W *et al*. Angiogenesis inhibitor-coated metallic stents in the porcine bile duct: prevention of benign reactive overgrowth. *Radiology* 1995; **197**: 695(P), 241.

55 Hehrlein C, Gollan C, Donges K *et al*. Low-dose radioactive endovascular stents prevent smooth muscle cell proliferation and neointimal hyperplasia in rabbits. *Circulation* 1995; **92**: 1570–1575.

56 Waksman R, Robinson KA, Crocker IR *et al*. Intracoronary radiation before stent implantation inhibits neointima formation in stented porcine coronary arteries. *Circulation* 1995; **92**: 1383–1386.

57 Schmitz-Rode T, Brune M, Hoffmeister K *et al*. High-frequency induction heating of stents: an approach to control intimal hyperplasia and tumour ingrowth. *Radiology* 1995; **197:** 1555(P), 382.

Index